Essential Skills Practice for OSCEs in Medicine

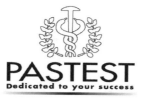

PASTEST
Dedicated to your success

Essential Skills Practice for OSCEs in Medicine

David R McCluskey

MD (Hons), FRCP, FRCPI, ILTM

Department of Medicine

Queen's University of Belfast

Belfast

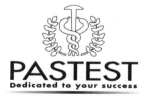

PASTEST
Dedicated to your success

© 2004 PASTEST Ltd
Egerton Court
Parkgate Estate
Knutsford
Cheshire
WA16 8DX

Telephone: 01565 752000

First published 2004

ISBN: 1 904627 38 2

A catalogue record for this book is available from the British Library.

The information contained within this book was obtained by the authors from reliable sources. However, while every effort has been made to ensure its accuracy, no responsibility for loss, damage or injury occasioned to any person acting or refraining from action as a result of information contained herein can be accepted by the publishers or authors.

Every effort has been made to gain consent to reproduce photographic material, x-rays and hospital documents. However if any have been inadvertently overlooked, the publisher will be pleased to make the necessary arrangements at the first opportunity.

PasTest Revision Books and Intensive Courses
PasTest has been established in the field of postgraduate medical education since 1972, providing revision books and intensive study courses for doctors preparing for their professional examinations.

Books and courses are available for the following specialties:
MRCGP, MRCP Parts 1 and 2, MRCPCH Parts 1 and 2, MRCPsych, MRCS, MRCOG Parts 1 and 2, DRCOG, FRCA, PLAB Parts 1 and 2

For further details contact:
PasTest, Parkgate Estate, Knutsford, Cheshire WA16 8DX
Tel: 01565 752000   Fax: 01565 650264
www.pastest.co.uk   enquiries@pastest.co.uk

Text prepared by Carnegie Book Production, Lancaster
Printed and bound in Europe by the Alden Group

Contents

History taking

Clinical signs

Clinical examination

X-ray

Data interpretation

Explanation/communication

Must-pass stations

Therapeutics and pharmacology

Acknowledgements

This book is dedicated to my sons Camin and Aled.

I wish to thank Kate Collins, John Collins and Kate Ritchie for helpful advice and suggestions, Mark Love for reviewing the radiology stations and David Gill for his expertise in preparing the visual aids. A very special thanks to Eveline Burns for her patience, help, encouragement and expert secretarial skills in the preparation of the text.

All photographic material, x-rays and hospital documents have been used with kind permission from the Royal Victoria Hospital, Belfast.

About the author

David McCluskey is Head of the Department of Medicine, The Queen's University of Belfast and Consultant Physician to the Royal Victoria Hospital, Belfast, with over 25 years' experience in undergraduate medical education. He introduced the OSCE form of assessment into the general medical course for 3rd year students in the Belfast Medical School and has extensive experience in constructing and marking this type of clinical examination as well as in acting as a simulated patient.

Other PasTest publications include – *Clinical Examination for Medical Students – A Hands-on Guide* and *100 Clinical Cases and OSCEs in Medicine* which was designed to be used in conjunction with this book.

Preface

Clinical assessment of undergraduate medical students and junior doctors in training is now commonly performed at clinical examination 'stations'. The Objective Structured Clinical Examination (OSCE) and the Practical Assessment of Clinical Examination Skills (PACES) are typical of these forms of assessment. This book consists of 143 typical OSCE stations together with model answers and can be used either to practice for this form of assessment or as a method of revision prior to taking other types of clinical examinations.

Further details of the clinical material on which the OSCE stations were based is available in the companion text, *100 Clinical Cases and OSCEs in Medicine*.

By working through the OSCE stations and becoming familiar with the case material, the format of the examination and the strengths and weaknesses of this form of assessment, the reader will not only improve their performance in clinical examinations but also develop and enhance the clinical skills that are essential for a good doctor.

Introduction

This book should be used in conjunction with other medical textbooks in order to revise and reinforce the knowledge gained through working through the OSCE stations. All of the stations contained within this text are based on a series of clinical cases which are commonly used in medical examinations and can be found in *100 Clinical Cases for OSCEs in Medicine*.

By working through these OSCE stations, acquiring a knowledge of the nature of this form of assessment and its inherent strengths and weaknesses, the reader will develop an understanding of what exactly examiners expect and of the ways in which he/she can display their competence more effectively.

The OSCE as a method of assessment

Objective Structured Clinical Examinations (OSCEs) were developed to address some of the problems associated with standard ward-based clinical examinations. The major criticism of these conventional examinations was lack of standardisation of the clinical material that was being used and, to a lesser extent, variation in examiners. For example, in the final clinical examination if you were fortunate enough to get a patient who was relatively young and articulate with a straightforward history, together with a benign examiner, the chances of getting a good mark were much greater than if the patient was frail, a poor historian with a complex history, and the examiner was a 'hawk' rather than a 'dove'.

The OSCE is constructed in such a way that all students cover identical or very similar clinical material and either have the same examiner or the marking system has been criterion-referenced and standardised so that there is no variation in examiners' marks. In this way all students get a fair, structured and objective test. Any differences in marks between students reflect differences in performance or competence in the tasks being assessed rather than variability in clinical material or examiner bias.

The examination usually takes the form of a circuit of 'stations' with each lasting five or ten minutes. At each station the student is asked to perform a task such as taking a clinical history, looking at an X-ray or investigation result and responding to a number of set questions, talking to a patient or simulated patient to explain a procedure or the examination of a system or part of a system. For an individual student the circuit usually consists of 10–20 stations and lasts for approximately 1–1½ hours. In order to complete an assessment of a cohort of students, several rounds of the circuit are usually necessary for the examiners and can take four to six hours in total.

One of the other perceived advantages of this type of examination is that it can process a fairly large number of candidates without causing major disruption to the clinical units. Because the OSCE is a circuit of stations it can be performed in a setting other than a ward and indeed is best done in a designated space such as an outpatient clinical area, day procedure unit or clinical skills area. This allows students and examiners adequate time and accommodation to perform the assessment without interruption or distraction.

The OSCE can be designed to test specific tasks deemed important by the examiners and is therefore less reliant on the clinical material present in a ward or hospital at the particular time of the examination.

Because the OSCE needs to be planned in advance, specifically to test certain skills, new methods of testing students have evolved. The 'simulated patient' is often used – these are actors or trained volunteers who can act the part of a patient with a specific history or problem which the student has to unravel, or a patient about to undergo a test or procedure and the student must explain the nature of the test and the implication of its findings. This works well for history taking and communication/explanation stations. At stations where physical examination is being tested, simulated patients may be used to assess competence at performing a systematic examination of a system or part of a system – for example, does the student perform a systematic, comprehensive and considerate examination of the abdomen, can the student test the function of all the cranial nerves? However, simulation does not work well in testing the ability of students to detect and identify abnormal clinical signs (see OSCE – strengths and weaknesses, pxviii) or for the examination of certain parts of the body – for example, it would be unreasonable to expect a simulated patient to allow 40 students to perform a rectal examination or urinary catheterisation, no matter how willing they were to help or how much money anyone was prepared to pay!

Alternative methods for testing some of these tasks have been developed. For example, the ability to detect and describe abnormal heart sounds and murmurs can be tested using audiotape recordings; abnormal retinal changes using photographs or slides; and examination of the rectum, scrotum, vagina and breast using anatomical models or mannequins, some of which can be modified in such a way that a variety of masses of differing size and consistency can be inserted to simulate the presence of a variety of tumours.

While the OSCE can be used to test knowledge, it is mainly used to test competence in vital clinical tasks – the ability to communicate with patients, take a history, examine in a systematic in a comprehensive manner, detect abnormality when present, interpret clinical, laboratory and radiological information, safely prescribe drugs, and safely perform those practical procedures which are essential for junior doctors.

OSCE planning and structure

An OSCE is usually planned by a group of clinical teachers who wish to test core knowledge and the full range of clinical skills.

Knowledge

Most medical schools use OSCE assessments in conjunction with other written forms of assessment, such as multiple choice or modified essay question papers. This is because there are only a limited number of stations in the circuit which are specifically designed to assess knowledge and the time at these stations is usually limited to five minutes. As a result it is not possible to assess a wide range or depth of knowledge at any one station.

For these reasons you can therefore be sure that the examiners will try to include the very important core topics in the curriculum, such as chest pain and/or shortness of breath as part of almost every diet of exams. Also, because time is limited, they will be looking for the key responses to be said first to indicate a good knowledge of the core topic being assessed. It is vital that you try to focus quickly on the important items of knowledge for each clinical scenario rather than worry about fine detail or 'small print' information.

Skills

It is agreed that certain key skills are vital for the practice of medicine and indeed the curriculum in most UK medical schools has been developed specifically to ensure that students have attained competence in these skills before graduation. The OSCE will be planned to test the full range of these skills and often an individual station will be designed to test more than one of these.

The key skills are:

1 **The ability to obtain and present a clinical history from a real or simulated patient.** In addition to assessing your ability to obtain all the important, relevant facts, the examiner will also be assessing your interpersonal skills, non-verbal communication, and your ability to 'manage' the interview – how well did you establish rapport with the patient, were you able to encourage a shy or reticent patient to talk, were you able to prevent a talkative patient from giving you irrelevant information, did you inspire trust and confidence etc?

2 **The ability to perform the physical examination.** There are three major objectives that the examiners will have at these stations:

    i   Do you know how to perform a comprehensive physical examination without causing distress or discomfort to your patient?

    ii   Is it obvious from your performance that you have had experience of performing this examination previously and therefore look and feel comfortable performing this task?

    iii Was the physical examination of such a standard that it would detect any abnormal physical finding that might be present?

3 **Communication skills.** Some of these have been mentioned earlier in the history taking section. Basically, the examiners will be looking for your ability to relate to and with your patient – how quickly and easily you establish rapport, establish appropriate eye contact, use both verbal and non-verbal cues to manage the interview so that information-gathering is efficient and comprehensive, yet allowing the patient an opportunity to talk, clarify and question. Avoiding medical terminology and jargon is extremely important as is talking to the patient in lay terms and at a level appropriate to the age, social group, IQ, educational level and personality of the patient.

4 **Therapeutics and pharmacology.** This subject is of vital importance in clinical practice and yet most medical schools which have developed an integrated systems-based course find that these important topics, which were conventionally taught in lecture courses, have less prominence in the curriculum. As a result, students feel less confident with their basic pharmacology knowledge and therapeutics skills. Unlike other university degrees, a medical degree brings with it a licence to prescribe potentially dangerous drugs and therefore certain key elements of pharmacology and therapeutics must be adequately assessed. These include pharmacokinetics and all aspects of pharmacodynamics. The basic principles of drug actions, the relationship between dose and response, drug absorption, metabolism and excretion, and of course all of the important therapeutic aspects including indications for the use of a drug, contraindications, side effects and interactions.

One of the standard methods of testing this knowledge is to use drug pre-scription charts which have a variety of drugs written out as if for a patient. These can be used to assess knowledge of drug dose, dosage regimes, drug interactions and practical aspects such as generic prescribing and contraindi-cations. Examples of how these are used are given in cases 127–143.

5 **X-rays.** All house officers are expected to be able to interpret commonly used X-rays, recognise major abnormalities and common acute medical disorders which can be revealed by this form of investigation. In the OSCE this knowledge is usually assessed at a fixed station where the student is presented with one or more X-rays and asked to identify the major abnormalities and give the most likely cause or a differential diagnosis. Sometimes this station can also be used to test other knowledge or skills. For example, if the X-ray is that of a patient with acute left ventricular failure the students may also be asked what treatment is required to treat the disorder – testing knowledge of therapeutics and pharmacology.

6 **Data interpretation.** It is often the pre-registration house officer who is the first person in the ward to see the results of the routine investigations which have been performed on the patients. It is essential that, before graduation, students are capable of recognising the presence of an abnormality, interpreting the common abnormalities in the full blood picture, biochemical analysis, bacteriology reports, pulmonary function tests and blood gas analysis, and of taking the appropriate remedial action which may be required. This is particularly important in the case of certain acute medical emergency situations, such as hyperkalaemia or acute renal failure. This is illustrated in cases 86-112.

Strengths and weaknesses

No single form of assessment is perfect and, like all others, OSCEs have some inherent strengths and weaknesses (see Table 1). But, overall, this form of assessment is a very powerful weapon in the examiner's armoury. Students can use their knowledge of the strengths and weaknesses to enhance their preparation for this type of examination. Because of the limited time to test knowledge at any given station, the student should concentrate on preparing answers which show that they have a good working knowledge of the common clinical features of those medical conditions which present commonly. The temptation to convey information about rare features should be avoided.

At all the stations with simulated patients, the examiners will be awarding marks for communication skills, style and professionalism. These marks can be easily 'earned' by concentrating on the 'General approach' section (pages xx–xxii).

Table 1 OSCE strengths and weaknesses

Strengths

- Objective test
- Standardised and fair
- Little chance of examiner bias
- Can be planned to test specific areas of knowledge and tasks
- Assesses both knowledge and skills in the context of a clinical setting
- Can test a wide range of skills
- Capable of assessing a large number of students
- No need to use patients in busy clinical wards
- Results and feedback can be obtained quickly
- Allows comparison of performance within a cohort of students
- Can identify weaknesses in individual students or in the group
- Ensures that all students are assessed on 'must-pass' topics

Weaknesses

- Cannot assess knowledge in depth
- Performance marks cluster around the mean value for the group of students
- Not suitable for assessing real patients who are very unwell
- Not suitable for assessing ability to detect abnormality
- Relatively easy to obtain marks with good communication skills and a professional approach
- Allocated time of five minutes per station is sometimes insufficient for taking a full history or completing a full examination, including hand-washing, etc

Marking schedules

The marking schedule that is used depends very much on the examiner's preference, and there is no standard scheme throughout all medical schools. Indeed some have dispensed with giving numerical marks altogether, and simply assess the performance as either unsatisfactory or satisfactory. However, most still have a fixation with assigning a mark, and examiners often spend many hours debating how many marks should be allocated to each station and the breakdown of marks within the stations. A typical mark-sheet that an examiner would use for a clinical examination station is shown opposite.

OSCE Station 9   **Clinical Examination – Neurology**

Introduction to student: Examine the power, tone and reflexes in both upper limbs of this patient

Student: Josephine Bloggs

	Not done, unsatisfactory	Satisfactory	Good
Marks to allocate	0	1	2
Student: Josephine Bloggs			
Student introduction			✔
Patient's name obtained		✔	
Consent given	✔		
Explanation of examination			✔
Limbs exposed			✔
Inspection for symmetry and wasting	✔		
Technique for testing power		✔	
Technique for testing tone			✔
Technique for testing reflexes		✔	
Intrinsic hand muscles tested	✔		
Additional marks for overall performance (maximum of 5)		3	
Total		14/25 Pass	

Comments/points for feedback or counselling:

Must obtain consent, inspect before proceeding to examination, and test muscles of the hands as well as the large muscle groups.

Some stations are classified as 'must-pass'. This means that no matter how well the student has performed in all other parts of the examination, failure at this station will result in failure of the whole OSCE. Must-pass stations include tasks, skills or knowledge that are deemed to be of vital importance for house officers and include the following topics:

1 basic life support

2 cardiac resuscitation (DC conversion)

3 death certification

4 management of anaphylactic shock

5 management of diabetic comas

6 management of acute haemorrhage.

These topics are covered in stations 121–126 in the must-pass section of this book. However, it is important to remember that if an examiner includes a topic as a must-pass station, they will have ensured that this topic has been covered in great detail as part of your undergraduate course. Teaching on the management of these conditions may vary from one medical school to another, and your response to the questions asked at these task stations should aim to satisfy the local examiner's protocols as accurately as possible.

General approach and how to maximise performance

Although it is impossible to pass an OSCE station with absolutely no clinical knowledge or ability, it is possible to register some marks and improve your score by paying attention to several simple techniques that are concerned with your general appearance and approach in those stations which have patients/simulated patients and examiners.

Dress and appearance

Although it may sound rather old-fashioned and fussy, there is no doubt that the way in which students dress and present themselves at the clinical stations does affect the mark they receive. This is not because examiners are likely to award more marks for someone with an attractive hairstyle or a trendy outfit. Rather it is because, like the general public, examiners expect young doctors in training to look as well as act like healthcare professionals. If you seem untidy, dirty or careless with regard to your appearance, this subconsciously suggests to patients that you may have a similar attitude to your work, which does not instil confidence and can impact on establishing a good doctor–patient relationship, which will often have to be demonstrated.

As a general rule, all students should wear clean white coats. Men should have neat hair, wear a shirt and tie, and avoid having a five o'clock shadow or 'stubble' beard. Women should wear their hair in such a style that it does not hang loose over the patient while they are carrying out a physical examination. All students should avoid chewing gum and wearing jeans or trainers. At all times they should avoid trendy language (phrases such as 'That's most helpful and interesting' are preferable to 'That's cool', etc).

Introduction

On entering a clinical station, it is important to act and behave as if you are the young doctor responsible for the patient's care. If an examiner is present, try to act as if they are not. Introduce yourself with your name and designated stage at medical school, and briefly inform the patient of the purpose of the station. For example, if you are entering a station where the instructions ask you to take a history from a patient (Mr Bloggs) who presents with shortness of breath and a cough, a good approach is to say 'Hello, Mr Bloggs. My name is Lesley Smith. I'm a fourth-year medical student. Would you mind if I talk to you for about five minutes and ask some questions regarding your recent illness?' While you are introducing yourself, shake hands with the patient to establish physical contact. If a chair is available, sit down to obtain the history – do not sit on the bed or stand over the patient like an inquisitor. Speak clearly and loud enough to avoid the patient having to ask you to repeat your questions. Further details of how to conduct the interview are given later in this book in the sections on history taking (stations 1 to 25) and explanation and communication (stations 113 to 120).

During the interview, avoid the use of medical terminology and jargon. As far as possible, use lay terms which members of the general public would understand. Always address the patient formally by their surname unless they are a child.

Be equipped

Be properly equipped for a clinical examination. Make sure that you have a pen as well as a watch with a second hand or digital second display so that you can record pulse and respiratory rates. A pen torch, stethoscope and tape measure are essential items of equipment which you should bring into the OSCE. If you have your own ophthalmoscope, patella hammer and/or blood pressure recording apparatus, this will impress the examiners. They will conclude that if you have gone to the trouble and expense of buying these items of equipment then you have probably gained some experience in their use. However, at stations where you are required to look at the fundi, test reflexes or check the blood pressure, the necessary equipment will be available to you. Before performing any physical examination or task on a patient, always explain what you are about to do and, if necessary, reassure the patient. For example, if you are asked to check the blood pressure, it is an excellent idea to ask the patient if they have ever had their blood pressure checked previously. If not, explain briefly how you are going to apply the cuff and inflate it, and inform them that they will feel some pressure where the cuff is applied and even some pressure building up in their hand and arm. Reassure them that the procedure will not be painful. Tell the patient to inform you if they find the procedure very uncomfortable or unpleasant, in which case you will stop.

Clarify the task

Occasionally when students enter a station the written or verbal instructions are unclear. Do not proceed until you have clarified exactly what is expected from you.

For example, if you enter a station and the examiner says 'Examine this patient's eyes', it may not be clear to you whether the examiner wants you to test visual acuity, fields of vision or extraocular muscle function, or simply to look at the eyes for evidence of underlying disease, such as exophthalmos, ptosis or xanthelasma. If on first inspecting the eyes there are no obvious clinical signs, ask the examiner to clarify the instructions by asking 'Do you wish me to test vision or eye movements?'

Summarise

At the end of each station where there is an examiner, when you have completed your task it is a good idea to summarise your findings. This is particularly important at history taking stations. When you have obtained the history, summarise it to the patient and ask them to confirm whether or not your version is accurate. Give them an opportunity to correct any misconceptions you may have or to add any additional information about which you may have forgotten to ask.

How to avoid failure

Students do not enter any examination with the intention of failing, and as a rule examiners are anxious that all students are successful. However, in the OSCE there are a number of ways to guarantee failure, and these must be considered so that they can be avoided. They include the following:

- being rude or inconsiderate to patients
- causing pain or severe discomfort
- suggesting the use of a drug at a lethal or dangerous dose, or a drug that is inappropriate or contraindicated
- being arrogant or self-opinionated
- failing to accept correction if one is wrong.

Thankfully it is rare for students to display such unprofessional and unacceptable behaviour in their assessments. However, many students throw away marks needlessly through less serious misdemeanours, such as the following:

- appearing in a dirty, untidy or inappropriate state of dress
- behaving in an inappropriate manner (eg joking or being too familiar with the patients)
- arriving at the examination ill-equipped (eg with no stethoscope or no watch)
- failing to introduce themselves to the patient
- failing to ensure that the patient is properly identified by asking their name
- using jargon and medical terminology which the patient is unlikely to understand
- failing to obtain consent before taking a history, performing an examination or carrying out a procedure
- failing to show adequate appreciation of the risks of cross-infection (eg not washing or disinfecting the hands between patients and/or procedures, not disposing of sharps safely).

Must-pass stations

Certain topics are deemed to be so important that they are prominent within the curriculum and extensively taught, and students are given clear warnings that they **will** appear in the assessment and an unsatisfactory performance **will** result in failure. The list of must-pass topics always includes basic life support, as it seems reasonable to expect all doctors to be able to sustain life until other help arrives. Many medical schools also include cardiac resuscitation (the knowledge and ability to recognise and treat life-threatening cardiac arrhythmias, including electrical cardioversion). Basic life support and cardiac resuscitation are covered in stations 121 and 122 in the must-pass section of this book, together with examples of what is expected in these must-pass stations.

Each medical school will only include such a station or stations if they are confident that all students have received adequate learning opportunities and teaching on these topics and the required protocols have been readily available for their students. Therefore there can be no excuse if students do not concentrate on these topics. It is a good idea to look carefully at your study guides in medicine or to ask your medical tutors to find out what the must-pass topics are and how they are managed and assessed. Some examples of other must-pass topics are included in stations 123–126.

History taking

Marking overall score for history taking and communication skills

Unsatisfactory	0	Major deficiencies in history taking
		Unsystematic approach to questioning
		Little concern for patient – used medical terms
		Failed to clarify
		Unprofessional
Below average	1	Minor deficiencies in history taking
		Unstructured approach to questioning
		Ill at ease with patient
Satisfactory	2	Competent history taking skills
		Adequate and systematic questioning
		Considerate to patient
		Good explanation of tests
Excellent	3	Highly competent history taking skills
		Very systematic questioning
		Well-organised sequence of investigation
		Professional and patient-centred

Communication skills

- Introduction
- Establishing nature of consultation
- Avoidance of medical terminology and jargon
- Summary of history
- Allowing patient to ask questions and clarify information
- Able to 'manage' dialogue (encourage reticent or control verbose historians).

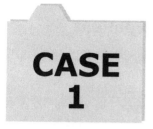

CASE 1

Chest pain

Instructions for student

This patient is complaining of chest pain. Take a history to determine the underlying cause, and inform the patient about the investigations that will be performed to confirm the diagnosis.

CASE 1

Instructions for examiner/simulated patient

You are a 45-year-old businessman who is experiencing central chest pain after meals and on exertion. You have smoked 40 cigarettes a day for 20 years, and have type 2 diabetes (diagnosed two years ago) that is well controlled by diet and a sulphonylurea drug. You have a positive family history of angina. The student must describe to determine increasing frequency and severity of angina pectoris in a patient with multiple risk factors.

Marking schedule

Chest pain:

- site
- character
- duration
- radiation
- precipitating factors
- aggravating factors
- relieving factors
- associated symptoms.

Risk factors:

- past history
- weight
- cigarette smoking
- family history
- diabetes
- hypertension
- cholesterol.

Investigations:

- exercise ECG
- coronary arteriography.

History taking and communication skills

Overall score:　　　　**0**　　　**1**　　　**2**　　　**3**　　　　**(please circle one)**

CASE
1

CASE 2

Chest pain and shortness of breath

Instructions for student

This patient was admitted with chest pain. Take a history in order to determine the most likely cause, and discuss the nature of the tests that will be performed to confirm the diagnosis.

Instructions for examiner/simulated patient

You are a 56-year-old schoolteacher who has a ten-year history of hypertension. You have had severe central chest pain for two hours and are beginning to feel short of breath. You are having an acute myocardial infarction and developing left ventricular failure, and you are experiencing nausea and sweating.

Marking schedule

Questions about pain:

- site
- severity
- radiation
- precipitating cause
- exacerbating factors
- relieving factors
- associated symptoms – shortness of breath, nausea, vomiting and sweating.

Questions about dyspnoea:

- orthopnoea.

Risk factors:

- past history of ischaemic heart disease
- hypertension
- diabetes
- cigarette smoking
- hypercholesterolaemia.

Investigations:

- ECGs – serial
- troponin.

History taking and communication skills

Overall score: 0   1   2   3   **(please circle one)**

**CASE
2**

CASE 3

Acute shortness of breath with chest pain

Instructions for student

This patient has recently returned from a holiday abroad. She complains of sudden-onset right-sided chest pain and shortness of breath. Take a history to determine the most likely cause of the patient's symptoms, and explain to her the nature of the investigations required to confirm the diagnosis.

Instructions for examiner/simulated patient

You are a young woman who has recently returned from holiday. This involved air travel for 19 hours. You have developed swelling of the left leg (deep vein thrombosis) followed by sudden onset of sharp localised pleuritic chest pain, shortness of breath (exercise tolerance 50 yards on the flat or ten stairs) and haemoptysis. You have no previous history of thromboembolic disease. You have been taking an oestrogen-containing oral contraceptive pill for two years. There is no significant past medical history, and you were in good health while on holiday.

Marking schedule

Questions to differentiate between pleurisy, pneumothorax and pulmonary embolus:

- sequence of symptoms
- site of pain
- type of pain
- associated symptoms (fever, dyspnoea, haemoptysis, sputum, deep vein thrombosis)
- past history
- drug history
- exercise tolerance.

Risk factors for deep vein thrombosis:

- immobility
- oral contraceptive pill
- family history of clots
- past history of clots.

Investigations:

- full blood picture, total and differential white cell count
- chest X-ray
- C-reactive protein
- ECG (S1, Q3, T3)
- D-dimer test
- ventilation-perfusion scan
- spiral CT scan
- pulmonary arteriography.

History taking and communication skills

Overall score: 0   1   2   3   **(please circle one)**

**CASE
3**

CASE 4

Increasing shortness of breath

Instructions for student

This patient has increasing shortness of breath. Take a clinical history to determine the most likely cause. Inform the patient of the investigations that you will arrange to confirm the diagnosis, and prescribe an oral drug therapy which would alleviate their symptoms.

Instructions for examiner/simulated patient

You are a 64-year-old with a past history of rheumatic fever and mitral stenosis, and underwent mitral valvotomy 40 years ago. Over the past six months you have developed increasing dyspnoea, four-pillow orthopnoea and paroxysmal nocturnal dyspnoea associated with a cough productive of frothy sputum. For two months you have had ankle oedema that is worse at the end of the day. In short, you have congestive cardiac failure. The student must take a clinical history, recommend a chest X-ray and prescribe a diuretic.

Marking schedule

Shortness of breath – established:

- severity (exercise tolerance)
- rate of progression
- orthopnoea
- paroxysmal nocturnal dyspnoea
- associated symptoms (cough and sputum production).

Ankle swelling – established:

- presence
- severity
- pattern – worse at night.

Reached diagnosis of left ventricular failure.

Reached diagnosis of congestive heart failure.

Explored past medical history:

- asked specifically about rheumatic fever
- asked about valve surgery.

Investigations:

- chest X-ray
- ECG
- echocardiography.

Treatment:

- appropriate oral diuretic drug.

History taking and communication skills

Overall score: 0   1   2   3   **(please circle one)**

**CASE
4**

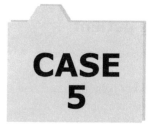

CASE 5

Shortness of breath and sputum production

Instructions for student

The patient at this station has shortness of breath. Take a clinical history to determine the most likely cause. Then inform the patient of the investigations that will be required to confirm the diagnosis and of the drug therapy which might be used to treat their condition.

Hint: Cough is present all year round. At present sputum is purulent and exercise tolerance is ten yards.

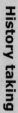

Instructions for examiner/simulated patient

You have chronic obstructive pulmonary disease (COPD) due to a 35-year history of smoking 40 cigarettes a day. At present you are extremely short of breath, with an exercise tolerance of ten yards on the flat or five stairs. You normally have a cough productive of mucoid sputum, but you also get frequent chest infections. You are having an acute exacerbation due to chest infection, with purulent sputum. You were employed by the Post Office for all of your working life. The student must take a clinical history to establish that you have chronic obstructive pulmonary disease and are having an acute exacerbation, and they must recommend appropriate investigations and treatment.

Marking schedule

Established current symptoms:

- shortness of breath
- cough
- purulent sputum
- fever
- absence of orthopnoea and paroxysmal nocturnal dyspnoea.

Ascertained:

- normal exercise tolerance
- present exercise tolerance characteristics
- normal sputum quantity and characteristics
- present sputum quantity and characteristics
- aggravating factors.

Past medical history:

- recurrent infections.

Occupational history.

Social history:

- housing (stairs)
- pets
- hobbies.

Drug therapy.

Diagnosed infective exacerbation of COPD.

Investigations:

- chest X-ray
- full blood picture and differential white cell count
- C-reactive protein
- sputum culture
- blood culture
- pulmonary function tests.

Treatment:

- broad-spectrum antibiotic
- inhaled bronchodilator therapy
- oral theophylline
- physiotherapy
- advice on smoking cessation.

History taking and communication skills

Overall score: 0   1   2   3   (please circle one)

CASE
5

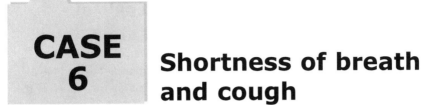

CASE 6

Shortness of breath and cough

Instructions for student

This 52-year-old patient has a history of shortness of breath and cough. Take a history to determine the nature of their symptoms, and suggest what investigations could be undertaken to determine the underlying cause.

Instructions for examiner/simulated patient

You are a 52-year-old dairy farmer who has experienced increasing shortness of breath for the past 18 months. You have a non-productive cough and have been feeling generally tired and lethargic. You used to work with mouldy hay and have farmer's lung. The student must take a clinical history to establish the nature of the patient's symptoms, and suggest appropriate investigations to confirm the presence of pulmonary fibrosis.

Marking schedule

Shortness of breath:

- severity (exercise tolerance)
- duration
- rate of progression
- orthopnoea
- absence of paroxysmal nocturnal dyspnoea.

Cough:

- presence of cough
- absence of sputum production.

Occupational history:

- established occupation as a farmer
- asked about exposure to mouldy hay.

Investigations:

- chest X-ray
- high-resolution CT scan of lungs
- pulmonary function tests (restrictive pattern)
- transfer factor (reduced)
- lung biopsy
- angiotensin-converting enzyme (ACE) – to rule out sarcoidosis
- antibodies to *Micropolyspora faeni* (thermophilic actinomycetes).

History taking and communication skills

Overall score: 0   1   2   3   **(please circle one)**

CASE
6

CASE 7

Shortness of breath and haemoptysis

Instructions for student

This patient has some shortness of breath and productive cough. Take a history to determine the underlying cause, and inform the patient of the tests that will be performed.

Instructions for examiner/simulated patient

You are a smoker of 40 cigarettes a day who previously worked in the building industry as a labourer and was exposed to asbestos. You have had a cough for 15 years, but recently noticed some blood in the sputum. You have anorexia, and have had weight loss of approximately half a stone (3.5 kg) in the past two months. Recently you have had three chest infections requiring hospital admission. Ask the student to tell you what tests will be performed. In summary, you have a bronchogenic carcinoma secondary to cigarette smoking and asbestos exposure, and require sputum cytology, chest X-ray, bronchoscopy and CT scan.

Marking schedule

Shortness of breath – established:

- severity (exercise tolerance)
- rate of progression.

Cough:

- nature of cough
- sputum production
- presence of haemoptysis
- change in character.

Associated symptoms – established:

- weight loss
- anorexia
- absence of night sweats
- asked about hoarseness.

Past history – established:

- recurrent chest infection – in the same lung
- smoking history
- occupational exposure to asbestos
- no history of tuberculosis.

Investigations:

- sputum cytology
- chest X-ray
- bronchoscopy with or without biopsy
- CT scan.

History taking and communication skills

Overall score: 0   1   2   3   **(please circle one)**

CASE 7

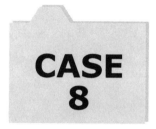

CASE 8

Shortness of breath and weight loss

Instructions for student

This patient has recently returned from India, where he has been working for the past two years. He has developed weight loss. Take a clinical history to determine the underlying cause, and inform the patient of the investigations which will be required.

Instructions for examiner/simulated patient

You have recently returned from India, where you have been working in an orphanage for two years. You have developed pulmonary tuberculosis and have the following classic symptoms:

- weight loss – two stone in six months
- night sweats
- cough with blood in the sputum
- anorexia and lethargy.

You are a lifelong non-smoker. The students must take a clinical history to determine the diagnosis. They have been informed that you have lost weight.

Marking schedule

Weight loss – established:

- degree of weight loss – two stone
- duration of weight loss – six months
- appetite change – anorexia
- no change in bowel habit
- no features of hyperthyroidism
- no features of malabsorption.

Respiratory symptoms – established:

- smoking history
- presence of cough
- presence of haemoptysis.

Constitutional symptoms – established:

- night sweats
- anorexia
- lethargy.

Asked about exposure to tuberculosis.

Asked about consumption of unpasteurised milk.

Investigations:

- chest X-ray
- sputum culture
- direct sputum microscopy.

History taking and communication skills

Overall score: 0 1 2 3 (please circle one)

CASE 8

CASE 9

Haemoptysis

Instructions for student

This patient has coughed up blood. Take a relevant history to establish the possible cause, and suggest what investigations would help to confirm the diagnosis.

CASE
9

Instructions for examiner/simulated patient

You are a 62-year-old who has developed haemoptysis. The student has been instructed to take a history and suggest investigations to identify the underlying cause. When giving your history, describe bruising easily, nosebleeds and bleeding from the gums, together with tiredness and lack of energy. You are to simulate a patient with chronic lymphatic leukaemia and thrombocytopenia.

Marking schedule

History to determine:

- haemoptysis – quality of blood
- weight change – none
- appetite – unchanged
- night sweats – absent
- non-purulent sputum production
- presence of epistaxis
- presence of skin bruises
- presence of bleeding gums.

Investigations:

- full blood count
- differential white cell count
- platelet count
- liver function tests
- coagulation screen
- bone marrow aspirate
- serum immunoglobulins.

History taking and communication skills

Overall score: **0**   **1**   **2**   **3**   **(please circle one)**

CASE
9

CASE 10

Dysphagia

Instructions for student

Please take a history from this patient, who is experiencing difficulty in swallowing. Also describe what investigations will be needed to confirm the diagnosis.

Instructions for examiner/simulated patient

You have been experiencing difficulty in swallowing for the past two months. Please describe symptoms consistent with a diagnosis of one of the following:

1   bulbar palsy
2   post-pharyngeal web
3   achalasia
4   oesophageal stricture
5   oesophageal carcinoma.

Marking schedule

Site of food sticking:

- high – oesophageal web
- mid-sternum – carcinoma
- lower sternum – carcinoma/stricture/achalasia.

Duration of symptoms:

- long – stricture/achalasia
- short – carcinoma/bulbar palsy.

Nature of symptoms:

- solids only – stricture/achalasia/web
- mainly liquids – bulbar palsy
- solids then liquids – carcinoma
- regurgitation of liquid through nose while swallowing – bulbar palsy
- recognition of undigested foods – stricture/achalasia.

Appetite:

- normal – web/stricture/achalasia
- poor – carcinoma.

Degree of weight loss (greater with cancer).

Duration of weight loss (shorter history with cancer).

Associated symptoms:

- neurological (bulbar palsy)
- pain (late feature of carcinoma)
- heartburn (stricture)
- anaemia/glossitis (web).

Investigations:

- oesophagogastroduodenoscopy (OGD with or without biopsy)
- barium swallow
- motility studies (oesophageal manometry).

History taking and communication skills

Overall score: 0   1   2   3   **(please circle one)**

CASE 11

Episodes of collapse

Instructions for student

This patient has had several episodes of collapse at home and at work. Take a clinical history to determine the nature of these events, and inform the patient of the investigations that will be performed to identify the cause.

CASE
11

Instructions for examiner/simulated patient

For the past six months you have been having episodes of collapse, both at home and at work. Some of these events have been witnessed. Between events you are asymptomatic. Please give a history consistent with one of the following:

1 drop attacks
2 transient ischaemic episodes
3 postural hypotension
4 vertebrobasilar insufficiency
5 Stokes-Adams attacks
6 aortic stenosis
7 epilepsy.

The student must take a clinical history and describe the appropriate investigations for confirming the diagnosis.

Marking schedule

Facts established by the student

Loss of consciousness or no loss of consciousness (drop-attack).

Prodromal symptoms:

- palpitations
- chest pain
- aura
- involuntary movements.

Precipitating causes:

- change of posture
- head movement
- exercise
- flashing lights
- infection/other illness.

CASE
11

Have events been witnessed?

Features of a typical episode.

Duration of the episode.

Symptoms between events.

Past medical history:

- head injury/surgery
- cardiac disease
- diabetes
- risk factors for stroke/transient ischaemic attack
- epilepsy
- rheumatic fever.

Drug history.

Investigations

For cardiovascular events:

- three- or five-day ECG monitoring
- echocardiography
- carotid and vertebrobasilar Doppler studies
- supine and standing blood pressure
- tilt-table blood pressures.

For neurological events:

- CT and/or MRI scan
- inpatient observation and EEG recording during an attack.

History taking and communication skills

Overall score: 0   1   2   3   **(please circle one)**

CASE
11

CASE 12

Swollen legs

Instructions for student

The patient at this station has some leg swelling which has developed within the past six weeks. Take a clinical history and inform the patient of the nature of the investigations that will help to determine the cause.

Instructions for examiner/simulated patient

The student must take a history and describe the investigations that will be required to identify the cause of your leg swelling. Please describe symptoms consistent with a diagnosis of one of the following:

1 deep vein thrombosis of one leg
2 right ventricular failure
3 nephrotic syndrome
4 cellulitis
5 ruptured Baker's cyst.

Marking schedule

Facts established by the student

One or both legs affected?

Extent of swelling.

Characteristics of swelling:

- colour of limb
- painful/pain-free
- variation during the day
- change in temperature
- tenderness.

Associated symptoms:

- fever
- malaise
- shortness of breath/chest pain
- joint pains
- periorbital swelling
- abdominal distension
- urinary symptoms.

CASE
12

Precipitating factors:

- periods of immobility
- trauma
- preceding infection.

Past history:

- deep vein thrombosis or pulmonary embolism
- cardiac disease (myocardial infarction or valve disease)
- respiratory disease
- renal disorders
- arthritis
- clotting disorders
- liver disease.

Drug history:

- oral contraceptive
- immunosuppressive drugs
- anti-inflammatory analgesics.

Investigations

Deep vein thrombosis:

- Doppler venogram
- coagulation studies.

Right ventricular failure:

- ECG
- echocardiography
- pulmonary function tests.

Nephrotic syndrome:

- serum electrolytes, urea, creatinine, total protein and albumin
- urinary protein estimation
- creatinine clearance test
- liver function tests
- autoantibody testing
- antistreptolysin-O titre.

CASE
12

Cellulitis:

- full blood picture and differential white cell count
- C-reactive protein
- blood cultures.

Ruptured Baker's cyst:

- rheumatoid factor
- arthrogram.

History taking and communication skills

Overall score: **0   1   2   3   (please circle one)**

**CASE
12**

CASE 13

Palpitations

Instructions for student

This patient has been experiencing palpitations. Please take a clinical history and inform the patient of the investigations that will be required to identify the cause.

Instructions for examiner/simulated patient

For the past three months you have been experiencing palpitations due to one of the following:

1 intermittent atrial fibrillation
2 ventricular ectopic beats
3 paroxysmal supraventricular tachycardia
4 self-terminating ventricular tachycardia.

Please give a history consistent with this diagnosis. The student must also inform you of the nature of the investigations which will be needed, namely ambulatory ECG monitoring and echocardiography.

Marking schedule

Onset (sudden or gradual).

Duration of event.

Rate (tachycardia or bradycardia).

Rhythm (regular or irregular).

Extra beats or missed beats.

Termination (sudden or gradual).

Associated symptoms:

- dyspnoea
- chest pain
- loss of consciousness
- faintness/dizziness
- flushing
- headache
- diuresis.

Past history:

- ischaemic heart disease
- valvular heart disease
- hypertension
- rheumatic fever
- alcohol abuse.

Precipitating factors:

- alcohol
- caffeine
- infection
- smoking cigarettes.

Drug history – cardiovascular drugs.

Investigations:

- resting ECG
- ambulatory ECG
- echocardiography.

History taking and communication skills

Overall score: 0 1 2 3 **(please circle one)**

CASE 13

CASE 14

Weight loss

Instructions for student

This patient has been referred by her family doctor. The patient's mother is very concerned about the degree of weight loss that has occurred. Please take a clinical history and describe the investigations that will help to identify the most likely cause.

Instructions for examiner/simulated patient

You are a 17-year-old girl with a history of rapid weight loss (two stones within three months). The student must take a clinical history and describe the investigations that will be required to make a diagnosis. Please give a history consistent with a diagnosis of one of the following:

1 anorexia nervosa
2 coeliac disease
3 Crohn's disease
4 thyrotoxicosis.

Marking schedule

Amount of weight loss.

Period of time over which weight loss has occurred.

Appetite.

Gastrointestinal symptoms:

- abdominal pain
- vomiting (spontaneous or self-induced)
- previous bowel habit
- present bowel habit
- steatorrhoea
- diarrhoea.

Associated symptoms:

- amenorrhoea
- skin rash
- uveitis
- tremor
- heat intolerance
- tiredness.

Dietary history – eating pattern (possibility of binge-eating).

Drugs – laxative use.

Psychological factors:

- self-image
- depression
- obsessional traits
- phobias
- preoccupation with body weight
- preoccupation with food.

Investigations:

- full blood picture
- biochemical profile for malabsorption
- small-bowel barium X-rays
- antigliadin and anti-endomysial antibody test
- thyroid function tests.

History taking and communication skills

Overall score: 0   1   2   3   **(please circle one)**

**CASE
14**

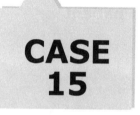

CASE 15

Weight loss and loss of appetite

History taking

Instructions for student

This patient has a history of significant weight loss (10 kg). Please take a clinical history and describe the investigations needed to determine the underlying cause.

CASE
15

Instructions for examiner/simulated patient

You are a 60-year-old painter/decorator with either:

1 carcinoma of the stomach, or
2 pancreatic carcinoma.

You have lost 10 kg in six weeks. Please give a clinical history consistent with this diagnosis, and ask the student to describe the investigations that will be necessary to reach a diagnosis.

Marking schedule

Duration of weight loss.

Change in appetite.

Abdominal pain:

- site
- character
- relieving factors
- radiation.

Vomiting with or without haematemesis and melaena.

Bowel habit – unchanged.

Jaundice.

Risk factors:

- cigarette smoking
- alcohol ingestion (pancreatic cancer)
- family history (gastric cancer).

Investigations:

- full blood picture
- liver function tests
- ultrasound scan of abdomen
- gastric – endoscopy and biopsy
- pancreatic – CT scan of abdomen, endoscopic retrograde cholangiopancreatography (ERCP).

History taking and communication skills

Overall score: 0   1   2   3   **(please circle one)**

CASE
15

CASE 16

Altered bowel function

Instructions for student

Please take a history from this patient who has altered bowel function, and inform him of the investigations which will need to be performed.

Instructions for examiner/simulated patient

The student has been asked to take a clinical history. They have been informed that you have altered bowel function. Please describe symptoms consistent with a diagnosis of either:

1 carcinoma of the colon, or
2 ulcerative colitis.

The student must also describe the nature of the investigations that will be required, namely colonoscopy with biopsy and barium enema.

Marking schedule

Normal bowel habit.

Present bowel habit.

Frequency of motions.

Consistency of motions.

Presence of blood.

Presence of mucus.

Abdominal pain:

- site
- character
- relieving factors.

Tenesmus.

Change in body weight.

Change in appetite.

For ulcerative colitis:

- malaise
- joint pain
- skin rash
- uveitis/scleritis
- positive family history.

For carcinoma of colon:

- positive family history
- personal or family history of colonic polyps.

Investigations:

- full blood picture
- liver function tests
- barium enema
- colonoscopy and biopsy.

History taking and communication skills

Overall score: 0   1   2   3   **(please circle one)**

CASE 16

CASE 17

Abdominal pain

Instructions for student

This patient has abdominal pain. Please take a detailed gastrointestinal history to determine the most likely cause.

CASE
17

Instructions for examiner/simulated patient

The student has been informed that you have abdominal pain, and must take a detailed history to determine the most likely cause. Please describe symptoms consistent with a diagnosis of one of the following:

1 gastric ulcer
2 duodenal ulcer
3 pancreatitis
4 gallstone colic
5 renal colic
6 Crohn's disease.

Marking schedule

Facts to be established about the pain by the student

Gastric ulcer:

- exact site – epigastric
- character – sharp
- severity – severe
- radiation – through to the back
- duration – minutes to hours
- precipitating/aggravating factors – food, aspirin, non-steroidal anti-inflammatory drugs (NSAIDs)
- relieving factors – antacids
- associated symptoms – weight loss, vomiting, haematemesis/melaena.

Duodenal ulcer:

- exact site – epigastric
- character – sharp
- severity – severe
- radiation – through to the back
- duration – minutes to hours
- precipitating/aggravating factors – hunger, aspirin, NSAIDs
- relieving factors – food, antacids
- associated symptoms – vomiting, haematemesis/melaena.

CASE
17

Pancreatitis:

- exact site – epigastric or central
- character – sharp
- severity – severe
- radiation – through to the back
- duration – hours
- precipitating/aggravating factors – large meal, alcohol
- relieving factors – leaning forwards
- associated symptoms – profuse vomiting.

Gallstone colic:

- exact site – upper abdominal
- character – colic
- severity – severe
- radiation – round to the right side of the back
- duration – variable
- precipitating/aggravating factors – fatty foods
- relieving factors – none
- associated symptoms – vomiting, flatulence, jaundice, dark urine, pale faeces.

Renal colic:

- exact site – renal angle
- character – colic
- severity – severe
- radiation – loin to groin
- duration – intermittent/variable
- precipitating/aggravating factors – none
- relieving factors – none
- associated symptoms – haematuria, vomiting.

History taking

CASE
17

Crohn's disease:

- exact site – central or right iliac fossa (RIF)
- character – crampy
- severity – moderate
- radiation – none
- duration – variable (hours to days)
- precipitating/aggravating factors – meals
- relieving factors – none
- associated symptoms – diarrhoea, constipation, weight loss, fever, rash, uveitis.

History taking and communication skills

Overall score: **0   1   2   3**   **(please circle one)**

**CASE
17**

CASE 18

Haematemesis

Instructions for student

The patient at this station has been vomiting. Please take a history to identify the most likely cause, and describe the main investigations that will be necessary to confirm the diagnosis.

Instructions for examiner/simulated patient

The student must take a detailed history and describe the investigations that will be needed. They have been told that the patient at this station is vomiting, but you should describe symptoms of haematemesis and other features consistent with a diagnosis of one of the following:

1 Mallory-Weiss tear
2 oesophageal varices
3 peptic ulceration
4 alcoholic gastritis
5 drug-induced gastritis.

Marking schedule

Duration of symptoms.

Appearance of vomitus:

- undigested food
- gastric contents
- bile.

Volume of vomitus.

Projectile or non-projectile vomiting.

Presence of blood or coffee grounds.

Total volume of blood lost (estimated).

Haematemesis with first episode of vomiting or subsequently.

Precipitating causes:

- dietary history, possible gastroenteritis
- drug history – especially aspirin, NSAIDs
- alcohol ingestion.

Associated symptoms:

- abdominal pain
- weight loss
- appetite
- constipation or diarrhoea.

CASE
18

Past history:

- chronic liver disease
- peptic ulcer
- pancreatitis
- gallstones
- previous gastrointestinal surgery
- other gastrointestinal disease.

Investigations:

- full blood picture, including platelet count
- prothrombin time
- liver function tests
- biochemical profile
- OGD.

Mallory-Weiss tear – vomiting gastric fluid followed by haematemesis (bright-red blood).

Oesophageal varices – past history of alcoholic liver disease. Sudden onset of large-volume haematemesis and melaena.

Peptic ulceration – dyspepsia typical of either gastric or duodenal ulcer, causing vomiting with haematemesis/coffee grounds and melaena.

Alcoholic gastritis – vague epigastric pain with coffee-ground vomitus togther with a history of **either** excessive alcohol ingestion **or** use of aspirin and/or NSAIDs for pain relief.

History taking and communication skills

Overall score: 0   1   2   3   **(please circle one)**

CASE 18

CASE 19

Jaundice

Instructions for student

This patient has developed jaundice. Take a history to determine the cause, and inform the patient of the nature of the investigations that will be performed to confirm the diagnosis.

Instructions for examiner/simulated patient

You have developed jaundice which is getting progressively worse. Over the past three weeks you have lost 3 kg in weight. The student has been asked to take a clinical history and describe the investigations needed. You will need liver function tests, viral hepatitis serology, abdominal ultrasound scan and CT scan of the abdomen. Please describe other symptoms consistent with a diagnosis of one of the following conditions:

1 viral hepatitis
2 alcohol-induced hepatitis
3 obstructive jaundice due to gallstones
4 obstructive jaundice due to carcinoma of the pancreas.

Marking schedule

Details established by the student

List of presenting complaints.

Duration of jaundice.

Associated symptoms:

- pain
- nausea/vomiting
- itching
- bruising easily
- urine colour
- colour of bowel motions
- ankle swelling
- weight change
- abdominal distension
- appetite
- vomiting/haematemesis.

**CASE
19**

Symptoms of anaemia.

Past history:

- anaesthetics
- blood transfusion
- exposure to hepatitis
- previous jaundice.

Drug history:

- paracetamol
- alcohol
- antibiotics.

Social history:

- occupation
- intravenous drug use
- sexually transmitted diseases
- foreign travel
- possible contact with rodents.

Investigations

Haematology:

- full blood picture and differential white cell count
- erythrocyte sedimentation rate (ESR)
- coagulation screen (especially prothrombin time).

Liver function tests:

- bilirubin
- aminotransferases (ALT and AST)
- alkaline phosphatase
- γ-glutamyl transpeptidase (GGT)
- serum albumin.

History taking

CASE
19

Viral hepatitis screening tests:

- serology and/or viral antigen tests
- ultrasound scan of abdomen
- CT scan of abdomen
- liver biopsy and histological examination.

History taking and communication skills

Overall score: **0**   **1**   **2**   **3**   **(please circle one)**

CASE
19

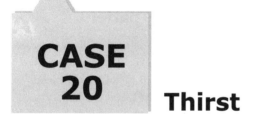

CASE 20

Thirst

Instructions for student

This patient is presenting with a severe thirst. Take a history to determine the cause, and inform the patient of the investigations that you plan to carry out to confirm the diagnosis.

CASE
20

Instructions for examiner/simulated patient

You have a history of thirst and polyuria for two months (drinking 8–9 litres of liquid each day, and taking drinks to bed with you because you waken at night feeling thirsty). You are passing a large volume of urine every 15–20 minutes. You have noticed tiredness and blurring of vision. After the student has taken the history, ask them to explain the nature of the investigations to be performed.

Please give a history consistent with a diagnosis of either:

1 diabetes mellitus, or
2 diabetes insipidus, or
3 hypercalcaemia secondary to multiple myeloma.

Marking schedule

Facts established by the student

Duration of symptoms.

History of initiating event:

- infection
- trauma
- surgery
- starting drug therapy.

Thirst awakening patient from sleep.

Severity of thirst.

Volume of fluid ingested each day.

Associated polyuria.

Volume of urine passed per day (approximate volume).

Associated symptoms:

- weight loss
- lack of energy
- altered visual acuity or field loss.

CASE
20

Past history:

- diabetes mellitus
- malignancy
- renal disease
- head injury
- metabolic disease
- pituitary tumours/surgery
- haematological disease
- respiratory symptoms.

Drug history:

- diuretics
- antidepressants
- antipsychotic drugs.

Family history:

- diabetes mellitus
- organ-specific autoimmune disease
- endocrine/metabolic disease.

Investigations

General:

- full blood picture
- electrolytes, urea and creatinine
- urine testing for protein, blood glucose.

For diabetes mellitus:

- fasting blood sugar
- glucose tolerance test.

For diabetes insipidus:

- serum and urine osmolality
- chest X-ray.

CASE
20

For hypercalcaemia due to multiple myeloma:

- serum calcium, phosphate, alkaline phosphatase and albumin
- skeletal X-rays
- chest X-ray
- isotope bone scan
- serum immunoglobulins and urinary Bence Jones proteins
- bone marrow biopsy.

History taking and communication skills

Overall score: **0**   **1**   **2**   **3**   **(please circle one)**

CASE
20

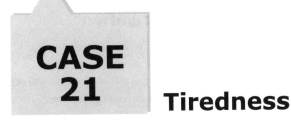

CASE 21

Tiredness

Instructions for student

This patient has been referred to the outpatient clinic complaining of tiredness. Please take a clinical history, and inform the patient of the various investigations you would recommend to identify the underlying cause.

CASE
21

Instructions for examiner/simulated patient

The student has been informed that you have been referred to an outpatient clinic complaining of tiredness. They must take a clinical history and inform you of the various investigations which will be performed to identify the underlying cause. Please describe symptoms consistent with a diagnosis of one of the following diseases:

1 anaemia secondary to dietary iron deficiency
2 pernicious anaemia with paraesthesia
3 anaemia secondary to haematological malignancy, with spontaneous bruising and petechiae.

Marking schedule

Clarified nature of symptoms:

- sleepiness/lassitude
- lack of energy
- muscle weakness.

Duration of symptoms.

Severity.

Rate of progression.

Precipitating cause.

Effect on activities of daily living.

Associated symptoms:

- weight change
- cold intolerance
- constipation
- appetite.

For a female patient – menstrual history.

Dietary intake – red meat, vegetables, dairy products.

Symptoms of overt blood loss:

- haematuria
- melaena or frank blood in motions
- haematemesis
- haemoptysis
- nosebleeds.

CASE 21

Symptoms of iron deficiency:

- glossitis
- brittle nails.

Symptoms of vitamin B_{12} deficiency:

- glossitis
- paraesthesia.

Symptoms of haematological malignancy:

- lymph node swelling
- bleeding gums
- petechial rash
- bruising.

Investigations:

- full blood picture
- differential white cell count
- iron, total iron binding capacity (TIBC) and ferritin
- serum vitamin B_{12} and folate levels
- thyroid function tests (T4 and TSH)
- serum immunoglobulins and urine for Bence Jones proteins
- biochemistry (sodium, potassium and calcium levels)
- urea and creatinine levels
- anti-parietal cell antibodies
- anti-intrinsic factor antibodies.

History taking and communication skills

Overall score:　　　**0**　　**1**　　**2**　　**3**　　**(please circle one)**

**CASE
21**

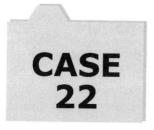

CASE 22

Headache

Instructions for student

This patient is complaining of headaches. Please take a history to determine the most likely cause, and inform the patient of the investigations which will be required to confirm the diagnosis and rule out other underlying abnormalities.

Instructions for examiner/simulated patient

At this history taking station the student has been informed that your presenting symptom is headache. The student must take a clinical history and inform you of the tests needed to identify the most likely cause and/or rule out other serious abnormalities.

Please describe symptoms consistent with a diagnosis of the following conditions:

1 tension headaches
2 migraine
3 temporal arteritis
4 raised intracranial pressure
5 meningitis.

Marking schedule

Exact site of pain.

Character (pressure, throbbing, tightness, stabbing).

Severity (on a scale of 0–10).

Onset – precipitating causes.

Exacerbating factors.

Duration/pattern.

Relieving factors.

Health between headaches.

Previous history of head or neck injury.

Previous history of hypertension.

Family history of renal disease.

Drug history – oral contraceptive pill in female patients.

Tension headache

Associated symptoms and factors:

- facial pain
- muscle stiffness in the neck
- stress
- occupation.

CASE 22

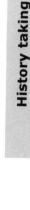

Investigations:

- X-ray of cervical spine
- MRI or CT scan of brain.

Migraine

Associated symptoms:

- paraesthesia or muscle weakness
- photophobia
- fortification spectra
- vomiting.

Investigations:

- CT scan of the brain is only needed if features are atypical or if the condition does not respond to appropriate therapy.

Temporal arteritis

Associated symptoms:

- blurring of vision
- stiffness of shoulder girdle muscles
- jaw claudication.

Investigations:

- erythrocyte sedimentation rate (ESR)
- temporal artery biopsy.

Raised intracranial pressure

Associated symptoms:

- vomiting without nausea
- neurological symptoms
- altered level of consciousness.

Investigations:

- CT or MRI scan
  Do not perform lumbar puncture.

CASE
22

Meningitis

Associated symptoms:

- fever
- skin rash
- photophobia
- neck stiffness
- vomiting.

Investigations:

- urgent CT or MRI scan followed by lumbar puncture for bacteriology, biochemistry and direct microscopy
- blood cultures.

History taking and communication skills

Overall score: **0**   **1**   **2**   **3**   **(please circle one)**

CASE
22

CASE 23 Confusion

Instructions for student

The patient at this station is confused. Please assess their mental state to determine whether this is an acute or chronic confusional state, and inform the patient of your decision.

Instructions for examiner/simulated patient

The student has been informed that you are confused. They must perform a mental state assessment to determine whether this is an acute or a chronic confusional state. If you are asked directly how long the condition has been present you should deny that you are confused at all, but otherwise behave towards and converse with the student in a manner consistent with either:

an acute confusional state (alcohol withdrawal state):

- no loss of short-term memory
- orientated in person
- disorientated in time and place
- visual hallucinations – insects on body
- agitated (eager to leave consultation), or

a chronic confusional state:

- loss of short-term memory
- retention of long-term memory (talk in detail about childhood)
- disorientated in time, person and place
- no hallucinations
- normal behaviour
- poor score for all Mini Mental State questions.

Marking schedule

Assessment of mental state

1 Orientation in time
2 Orientation in person
3 Orientation in place
4 Test of short-term memory
5 Test of intellectual ability (eg serial sevens)
6 Test of language:

- naming objects
- repeating a phrase
- reading an instruction and performing a task
- performing a simple task

7 Visuospatial task (eg drawing geometric symbol)
8 Test of long-term/past memory.

CASE
23

Acute confusional state:

- 1–3 very poor
- 8 poor
- visual hallucinations
- agitation.

Chronic confusional state:

- 1–7 poor
- 8 excellent.

History taking and communication skills

Overall score: **0**   **1**   **2**   **3**   **(please circle one)**

CASE 24

Joint pain

Instructions for student

This patient has joint pains. Take a history to determine the features, and explain to the patient what investigations will be performed.

Instructions for examiner/simulated patient

The student has been informed that you have joint pains. They have been asked to take a history and to describe the investigations needed to make a diagnosis.

Please describe symptoms consistent with a diagnosis of systemic lupus erythematosus, including the following:

- morning stiffness of hands
- intermittent attacks of hot, swollen, tender joints
- mouth ulceration
- photosensitive skin rash on the face
- previous episodes of pleurisy
- Raynaud's phenomenon.

Then ask the student what they think is the most likely diagnosis.

Marking schedule

Duration of symptoms.

Joints affected.

Characteristics of joints:

- hot
- swollen
- stiff
- tender
- loss of function
- intermittent attacks
- no residual deformity.

Presence of mouth ulceration.

No discoid lupus rash.

Photosensitivity of skin on face.

No alopecia.

Raynaud's phenomenon.

Episodes of pleurisy in the past.

No previous pericarditis or peritonitis.

No past history of deep vein thrombosis or pulmonary embolism.

**CASE
24**

Drug history – in the case of the female patient, asked specifically about oral contraceptive use.

Investigations:

- full blood picture
- erythrocyte sedimentation rate (ESR)
- antinuclear antibody
- anti-double-stranded DNA antibody test
- complement levels
- serum electrolytes, urea and creatinine
- 24-hour urinary protein excretion
- creatinine clearance test.

Diagnosis of systemic lupus erythematosus.

History taking and communication skills

Overall score: **0**   **1**   **2**   **3**   **(please circle one)**

CASE 24

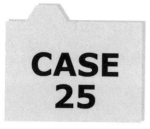

CASE 25

Depression

Instructions for student

This patient took an overdose of paracetamol (15 x 500 mg tablets) three days ago. The overdose was managed correctly. Please assess the patient and complete the form below to indicate your findings and opinion. Then give the form to the patient or examiner.

Patient questionnaire

Mental State Assessment Form

1 Appearance and behaviour

2 Speech

3 Affect (mood)

4 Thought content

5 Does the patient have abnormal perceptions?
         Yes / No (please circle)

6 Cognitive state

7 What is the diagnosis?

8 Can the patient be discharged today?
         Yes / No (please circle)

9 What are the risks of a repeat attempt at self-harm?
         Low / Moderate / High (please circle one answer)

10 Name two classes of drugs that might be considered for this patient.

CASE 25

Instructions for examiner/simulated patient

You were admitted three days ago after a drug overdose with paracetamol. The student has been asked to determine your mental state. Please respond to their questions on the assessment form provided (which the student must complete) as indicated below:

- Admit to feeling depressed and hopeless.
- You have been divorced for two years and feel lonely.
- You live alone in a flat and rarely cook.
- You were made redundant six months ago with no prospect of work – this is a preoccupation with you.
- You drink at least 15 units of alcohol every day, usually alone in your flat.
- You awaken at 3 am and are unable to get back to sleep.
- You feel sure that you have cancer of the lung, and are preoccupied with this thought.
- This is your first overdose, but you have had ideas of suicide for three months.
- If asked, admit that you would attempt suicide again.
- You have had no hallucinations or illusions, and no feelings of depersonalisation.
- You are well orientated, with normal short- and long-term memory.

CASE 25

Marking schedule

Mental State Assessment Form

1 Appearance and behaviour:
- underactive
- untidy dress
- unco-operative.

2 Speech:
- slow
- quietly spoken.

3 Affect (mood):
- looks and acts depressed
- admits to depression.

4 Thought content:
- thoughts of suicide
- preoccupied with health
- hopelessness – no prospect of work.

5 Does the patient have abnormal perceptions?
   No.

6 Cognitive state:
- orientation (well orientated)
- memory (good short- and long-term memory).

7 What is the diagnosis?
   Reactive depression.

8 Can the patient be discharged today?
   No.

9 What are the risks of a repeat attempt at self-harm?
   High.

10 Name two classes of drugs that might be considered for this patient:
- tricyclic antidepressants
- serotonin re-uptake inhibitors.

History taking and communication skills

Overall score: 0 1 2 3 **(please circle one)**

CASE 25

Clinical signs

CASE 26

General inspection: eyes

1 What name is given to the skin lesions present?

2 What other abnormality is present?

3 What blood test would confirm the diagnosis?

4 What medical disorders are associated with this appearance?

5 How is this condition managed?

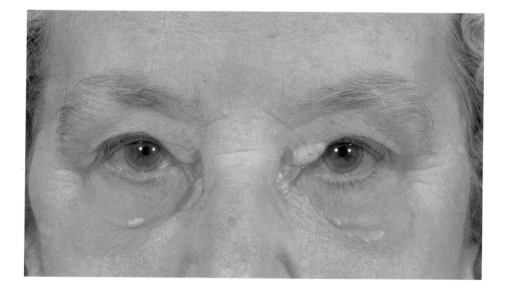

Answers

1 What name is given to the skin lesions present?

Xanthelasma.

2 What other abnormality is present?

Corneal arcus.

3 What blood test would confirm the diagnosis?

Fasting lipids/cholesterol.

4 What medical disorders are associated with this appearance?

- *Hypothyroidism*
- *Familial hyperlipidaemia/familial hypercholesterolaemia*
- *Diabetes mellitus*
- *Hypertension*
- *Ischaemic heart disease*
- *Primary biliary cirrhosis*
- *Nephrotic syndrome.*

5 How is this condition managed?

- *Dietary advice – low-fat diet*
- *Drugs – statin.*

CASE 26

CASE 27

General inspection: face (1)

This woman was asked to show her teeth.

1 What abnormality is present?

2 What else would you ask the patient to do to determine the nature of the abnormality?

3 List the possible causes.

4 How can one differentiate between lesions of the upper and lower motor neurone pathway in this condition?

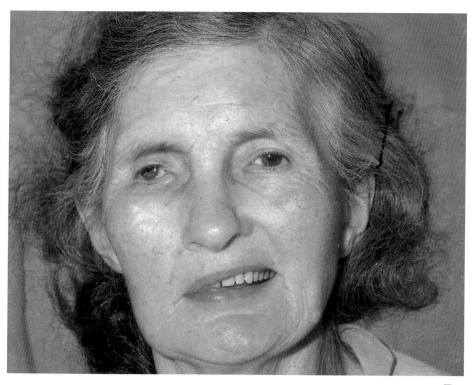

Answers

1 What abnormality is present?

Right facial nerve palsy.

2 What else would you ask the patient to do to determine the nature of the abnormality?
- *Raise eyebrows/wrinkle forehead*
- *Blow out cheeks*
- *Close eyes tight*
- *Check power in limbs.*

3 List the possible causes.
- *Bell's palsy*
- *Cerebrovascular accident*
- *Trauma/surgery*
- *Tumour.*

4 How can one differentiate between lesions of the upper and lower motor neurone pathway in this condition?

Movement of the forehead is absent in lower motor neurone lesions.

CASE
27

CASE 28

General inspection: face (2)

This woman has a history of gradually progressive shortness of breath.

1 What cardiac disorder would you consider?

2 What would the classic findings be on auscultation of the heart? Please comment on the first heart sound and on each phase of the cardiac cycle in sequence.

3 What rhythm disorder commonly occurs as a complication?

4 What investigations would confirm the presence of the cardiac involvement?

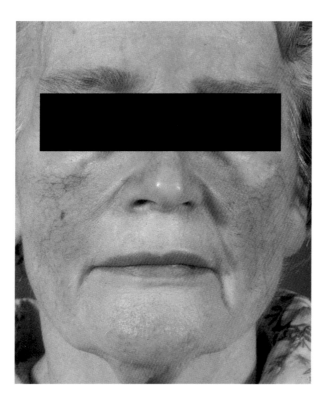

Answers

1 What cardiac disorder would you consider?
   Mitral stenosis.

2 What would be the classic findings on auscultation of the heart? Please comment on the first heart sound and on each phase of the cardiac cycle in sequence.
   - *Loud first heart sound*
   - *Normal second heart sound, opening snap*
   - *Mid-diastolic murmur*
   - *Presystolic accentuation (if patient is in sinus rhythm).*

3 What rhythm disorder commonly occurs as a complication?
   Atrial fibrillation.

4 What investigations would confirm the presence of the cardiac involvement?
   - *Echocardiography*
   - *ECG*
   - *Cardiac catheterisation.*

Clinical signs

CASE 28

CASE 29

General inspection: face (3)

This young woman complains of episodes of painless swelling of the soft tissues of the face, especially the periorbital area, lips and tongue.

1 What name is given to this condition?

2 What skin rash is it often associated with?

3 List three possible causes.

4 If several members of the patient's family were affected, what condition would you suspect?

5 What blood test would confirm this diagnosis in the family?

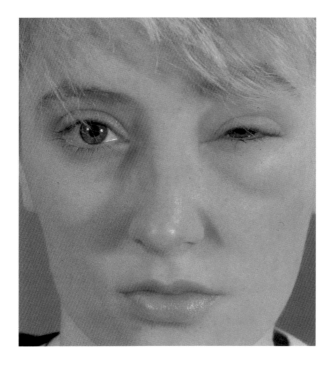

Clinical signs

Answers

1 What name is given to this condition?
    Angio-oedema.

2 What skin rash is it often associated with?
    Urticaria.

3 List three possible causes.
    - *Idiopathic*
    - *Allergy*
    - *Physical cause (light, cold, pressure, water).*

4 If several members of the patient's family were affected, what condition would you suspect?
    Hereditary angio-oedema.

5 What blood test would confirm this diagnosis in the family?
    C1 esterase inhibitor – low level.

Clinical signs

CASE 29

CASE 30

General inspection: face and hands (1)

1 On inspection of this photograph, what is the most likely diagnosis?

2 What is the underlying cause?

3 List three medical disorders which may complicate this condition.

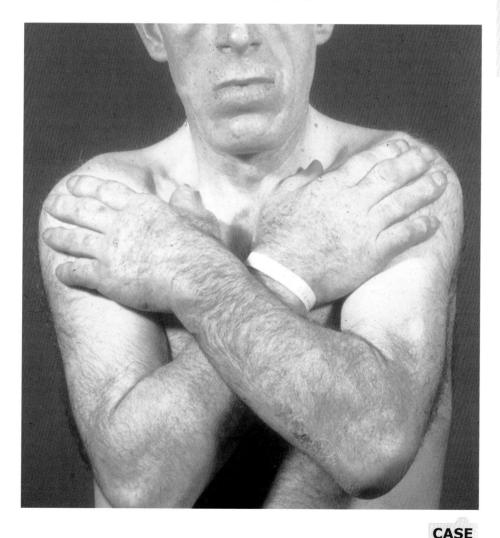

Answers

1 On inspection of this photograph, what is the most likely diagnosis?
Acromegaly.

2 What is the underlying cause?
Excess growth hormone production from pituitary adenoma.

3 List three medical disorders which may complicate this condition.
- *Diabetes*
- *Bitemporal hemianopia*
- *Cardiac failure*
- *Hypertension*
- *Arthropathy*
- *Renal stones*
- *Carpal tunnel syndrome.*

Clinical signs

CASE 30

CASE 31

General inspection: face and hands (2)

This woman has a ten-year history of Raynaud's phenomenon.

1 What diagnosis would you consider?

2 List four classic features of the condition.

3 What blood tests may help to confirm the diagnosis?

4 The patient describes increasing shortness of breath. What two respiratory complications can occur?

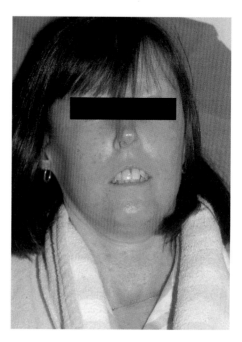

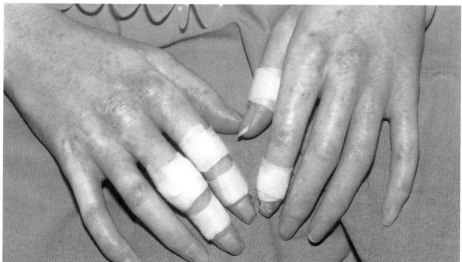

CASE 31

Answers

1 What diagnosis would you consider?
   Scleroderma/CREST syndrome.

2 List four classic features of the condition.
   - *Sclerodactyly*
   - *Telangiectasia*
   - *Dysphagia*
   - *Subcutaneous calcification*
   - *Tethering of skin over the forehead and nose*
   - *Microstomia*
   - *Pulmonary fibrosis.*

3 What blood tests may help to confirm the diagnosis?
   - *Anticentromere antibodies*
   - *Anti-ScL-70 antibodies.*

4 The patient describes increasing shortness of breath. What two respiratory
   complications can occur?
   - *Pulmonary fibrosis*
   - *Aspiration pneumonia.*

**CASE
31**

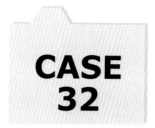

CASE 32

General inspection

This young man has a history of spontaneous pneumothorax.

1 What condition would you consider on general inspection?

2 List three complications which can occur.

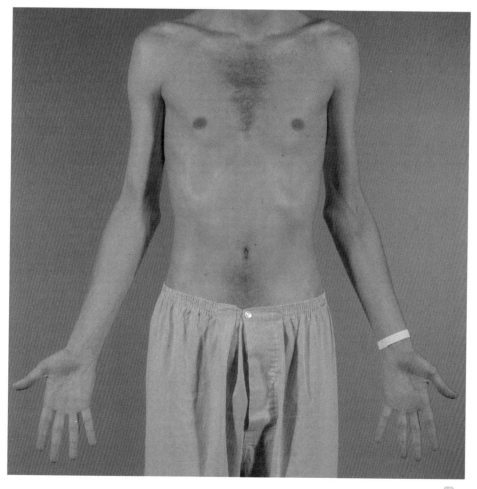

CASE 32

Answers

1 What condition would you consider on general inspection?
   Marfan's syndrome.

2 List three complications which can occur.
   - *Dislocated lens*
   - *Aortic dissection*
   - *Mitral valve prolapse*
   - *Pneumothorax.*

CASE
32

CASE 33

General inspection: neck

Clinical signs

This woman has a four-week history of headache, loss of appetite and 2-kg weight loss. On examination she has reduced expansion of the right side of the chest. There is reduced air entry and a late expiratory wheeze over the left upper lobe.

1 What abnormalities are seen on examination of this photograph?

2 What differential diagnosis would you consider if you saw this appearance?

3 What is the most likely cause in a patient with this history?

4 What investigations will confirm the diagnosis?

5 What clinical signs would you specifically look for on examination of the patient's face?

6 Apart from analgesic drugs, what treatment can be given to relieve the headache?

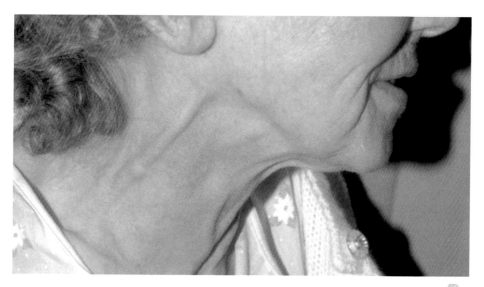

CASE 33

Answers

1 What abnormalities are seen on examination of this photograph?

Distension of the jugular venous system.

2 What differential diagnosis would you consider if you saw this appearance?
- *Superior vena caval obstruction*
- *Right ventricular failure*
- *Pericardial effusion*
- *Constrictive pericarditis.*

3 What is the most likely cause in a patient with this history?

Superior vena caval obstruction due to a lung tumour.

4 What investigations will confirm the diagnosis?
- *Chest X-ray*
- *CT scan of the chest*
- *Sputum cytology.*

5 What clinical signs would you specifically look for on examination of the patient's face?
- *Miosis*
- *Anhidrosis*
- *Ptosis*
- *Apparent enophthalmos.*

6 Apart from analgesic drugs, what treatment can be given to relieve the headache?

Radiotherapy to shrink the tumour.

CASE 33

CASE 34

Sputum samples

These sputum samples are from two different patients.

1 Describe each.

2 What is the most likely cause of each?

3 If one of the samples was bloodstained, which would be more likely to be associated with a lung tumour?

4 What is the most common underlying cause of the type of sputum marked 'B'?

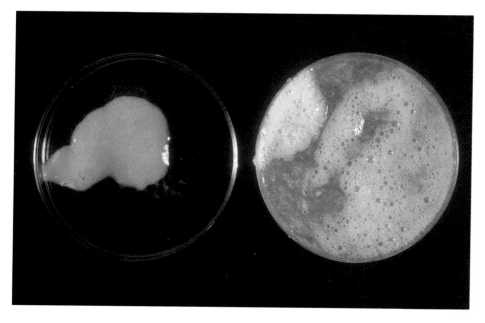

A   **B**

CASE
34

Answers

1 Describe each.
>   A *Thick, green, purulent*
>
>   B *White, frothy.*

2 What is the most likely cause of each?
>   A *Chest infection*
>
>   B *Pulmonary oedema.*

3 If one of the samples was bloodstained, which would be more likely to be associated with a lung tumour?
>   *'A' would be more likely to be associated with a lung tumour.*

4 What is the most common underlying cause of the type of sputum marked 'B'?
>   *Left ventricular failure.*

CASE 34

CASE 35

Skin lesions with blood pressure measurement

This woman developed these skin lesions only while her blood pressure was being recorded. The lesions were only present below the cuff.

1 What is the name given to these skin lesions?

2 What is the mechanism that causes this to happen?

3 What name is given to this procedure when it is used as a diagnostic test?

4 What haematological investigations will help to determine the cause?

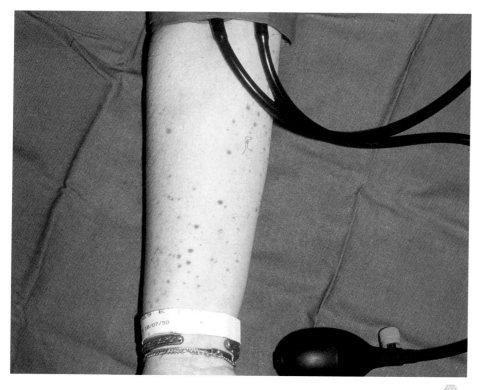

Answers

1 What is the name given to these skin lesions?
   Petechiae.

2 What is the mechanism that causes this to happen?
   Bleeding from vessels under increased pressure.

3 What name is given to this procedure when it is used as a diagnostic test?
   Hess test.

4 What haematological investigations will help to determine the cause?
   - *Platelet count*
   - *Platelet function tests.*

Clinical signs

CASE
35

CASE 36

Skin lesions (1)

1 What name is given to these skin lesions?

2 List four possible causes.

3 What investigations would be appropriate to rule out an underlying medical cause?

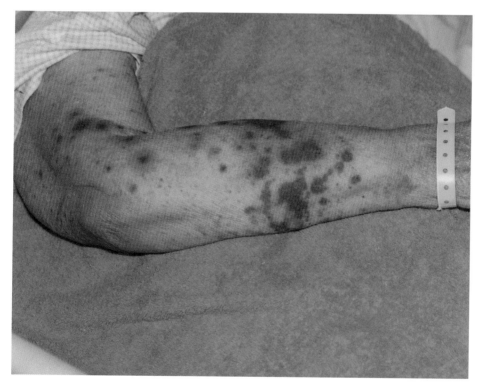

Answers

1 What name is given to these skin lesions?
> *Purpura.*

2 List four possible causes.
- *Steroids*
- *Warfarin*
- *Thrombocytopenia*
- *Liver failure*
- *Senility*
- *Bleeding disorder*
- *Vitamin C deficiency (scurvy).*

3 What investigations would be appropriate to rule out an underlying medical cause?
- *Platelet count*
- *Platelet function tests*
- *Coagulation screen*
- *Liver function tests.*

Clinical signs

CASE 36

CASE 37

Skin lesions (2)

This elderly man has a 30-year history of non-itchy skin lesions all over the body.

1 What is the diagnosis?

2 The patient has lower back pain. What joint condition may complicate this disorder?

3 List four types of drug therapy that can be used to treat this rash.

4 What other form of treatment is used for this condition?

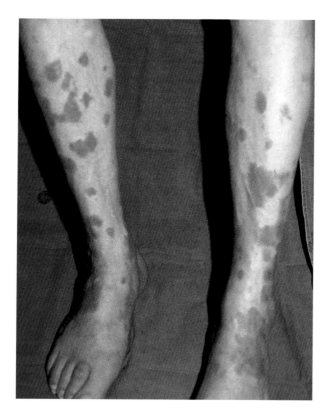

CASE
37

Answers

1 What is the diagnosis?

Psoriasis.

2 The patient has lower back pain. What joint condition may complicate this disorder?

- *Psoriatic arthropathy*
- *Sacroiliitis.*

3 List four types of drug therapy that can be used to treat this rash.

- *Coal tar preparations*
- *Steroids*
- *Retinoids*
- *Cytotoxic drugs.*

4 What other form of treatment is used for this condition?

Phototherapy – psoralen plus ultraviolet A radiation (PUVA).

Clinical signs

CASE
37

CASE 38

Skin lesions (3)

This patient has developed red, painful, tender lesions of the lower legs.

1 What is the diagnosis?

2 List four common causes.

3 What is the treatment?

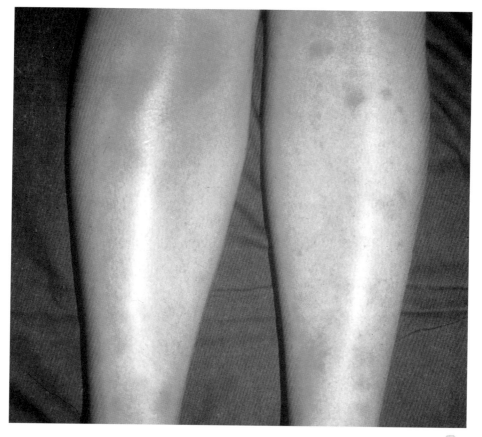

Answers

1 What is the diagnosis?

   Erythema nodosum.

2 List four common causes.
   - *Post-streptococcal*
   - *Sarcoid*
   - *Drugs – sulphonamides/oral contraceptive pill*
   - *Inflammatory bowel disease.*

3 What is the treatment?
   - *Treat underlying cause*
   - *Bedrest*
   - *Non-steroidal anti-inflammatory drugs/steroids.*

CASE
38

CASE 39

Skin lesions (4)

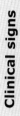

This woman has had a facial rash for six months, and also has severe joint pain with swelling and stiffness of the small joints of both hands.

1 What diagnosis would you consider?

2 List four other features of this condition.

3 What blood tests would confirm the diagnosis?

4 What is the usual cause of death in this disorder?

5 What treatment is used to control major organ involvement?

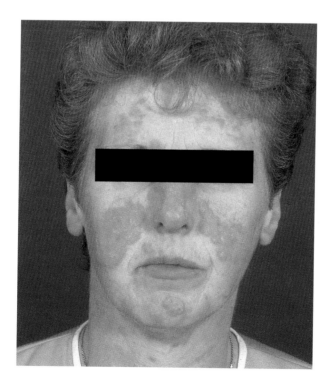

CASE
39

Answers

1 What diagnosis would you consider?
   Systemic lupus erythematosus.

2 List four other features of this condition.
   - *Mouth ulcers*
   - *Raynaud's phenomenon*
   - *Serositis*
   - *Alopecia*
   - *Digital ischaemia*
   - *Vasculitic rash*
   - *Neurological symptoms*
   - *Haematological disorder*
   - *Renal disease*
   - *False-positive serology for syphilis*
   - *Immunological abnormality.*

3 What blood tests would confirm the diagnosis?
   - *Antinuclear antibody*
   - *Anti-double-stranded DNA antibody test.*

4 What is the usual cause of death in this disorder?
   Renal failure.

5 What treatment is used to control major organ involvement?
   Corticosteroids and immunosuppressive drugs.

CASE
39

CASE 40

Skin lesions (5)

This woman has a history of diarrhoea with blood and mucus in the stools.

1 What name is given to this skin lesion?

2 What is the likely cause of the patient's gastrointestinal symptoms?

3 What investigations would be useful to confirm the diagnosis?

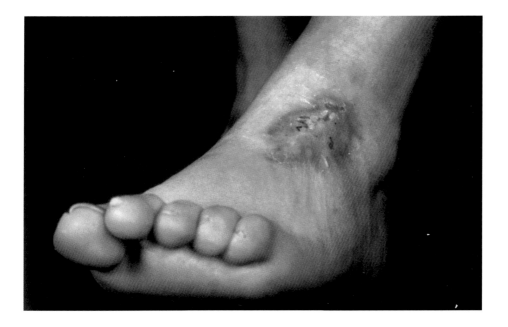

Answers

1 What name is given to this skin lesion?
   Pyoderma gangrenosum.

2 What is the likely cause of the patient's gastrointestinal symptoms?
   Ulcerative colitis.

3 What investigations would be useful to confirm the diagnosis?
   - *Barium X-ray of the large bowel*
   - *Colonoscopy with biopsy to show histological features.*

Clinical signs

CASE
40

CASE 41

Skin lesions (6)

This patient gives a history of right-sided chest pain for four days, followed by the development of this rash.

1 What is the diagnosis?

2 What organism is associated with this rash?

3 What may cause this condition to occur?

4 What treatment is given for the rash?

5 What treatment is given for the severe pain which may occur during the rash and after it resolves?

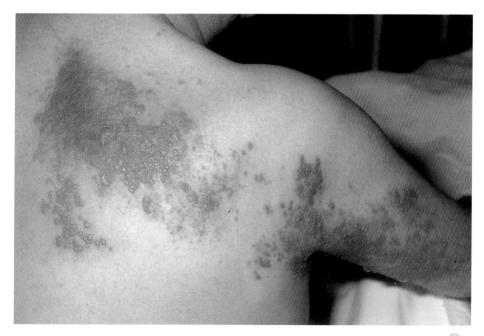

CASE 41

Answers

1 What is the diagnosis?

Herpes zoster/shingles.

2 What organism is associated with this rash?

Varicella zoster (DNA) virus.

3 What may cause this condition to occur?
- *AIDS or other immunodeficiency states*
- *Immunosuppressive drugs*
- *Underlying malignancy*
- *Steroid therapy.*

4 What treatment is given for the rash?
- *Analgesia*
- *Aciclovir.*

5 What treatment is given for the severe pain which may occur during the rash and after it resolves?
- *Tricyclic antidepressants*
- *Carbamazepine*
- *Gabapentin.*

CASE 41

CASE 42

Skin lesions (7)

The skin lesion shown developed on this woman's leg two months ago. There is no history of trauma. On examination of the abdomen the liver is found to be 5 cm enlarged, with an irregular surface.

1 What is the most likely diagnosis for the skin lesion?

2 What is causing the liver enlargement?

3 What factors predispose to the development of this condition?

4 What is causing the discoloration of the blood vessel seen to the right of the skin lesion?

5 What forms of treatment are used for this condition?

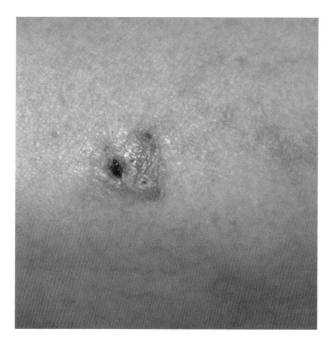

Answers

1 What is the most likely diagnosis for the skin lesion?
    Malignant melanoma.

2 What is causing the liver enlargement?
    Liver metastases.

3 What factors predispose to the development of this condition?
    - *Sunlight exposure*
    - *Genetic susceptibility*
    - *Multiple pigmented naevi.*

4 What is causing the discoloration of the blood vessel seen to the right of the skin lesion?

    Direct spread of pigmented tumour into the vessel wall.

5 What forms of treatment are used for this condition?
    - *Deep and wide surgical resection of regional lymph nodes*
    - *Immunotherapy.*

CASE 42

CASE 43

Skin lesions (8)

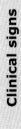

This boy has had a skin rash since infancy. It is itchy and occasionally bleeds.

1 Describe the distribution of the rash and its morphological features.

2 What is the most likely diagnosis?

3 What other symptoms not related to his skin might the patient have?

4 What blood test would be abnormal?

5 List three forms of treatment which are used for this rash.

6 Of 100 patients with this disorder, approximately how many will continue to have a troublesome rash in adult life?

   2   10   25   45   75   (please circle the correct answer)

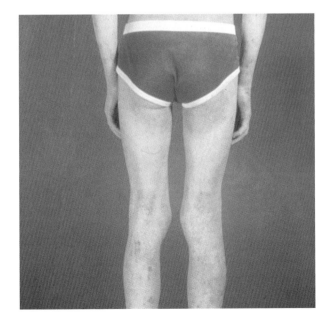

CASE
43

Answers

1 Describe the distribution of the rash and its morphological features.
- *Flexural*
- *Erythematous, ichthyotic.*

2 What is the most likely diagnosis?
  Atopic eczema.

3 What other symptoms not related to his skin might the patient have?
- *Allergic rhinitis (hay fever)*
- *Allergic conjunctivitis (hay fever)*
- *Asthma.*

4 What blood test would be abnormal?
- *Raised serum IgE*
- *Positive RAST to common antigens.*

5 List three forms of treatment which are used for this rash.
- *Emollients*
- *Topical steroids*
- *Occlusive dressings*
- *Antigen avoidance measures.*

6 Of 100 patients with this disorder, approximately how many will continue to have a troublesome rash in adult life?

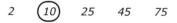

   2   (10)   25   45   75

CASE
43

CASE 44

Skin lesions (9)

This photograph was taken of the lower chest/upper abdomen of a 20-year-old man.

1 Describe the skin abnormality seen here.

2 What is the most likely diagnosis?

3 On which structures do these lesions develop?

4 The condition is confined to the skin only.

      True   False   (circle the correct answer)

5 What is the usual pattern of inheritance?

6 What other tumours can occur in association with this disorder?

7 What other medical disorders are associated with this condition?

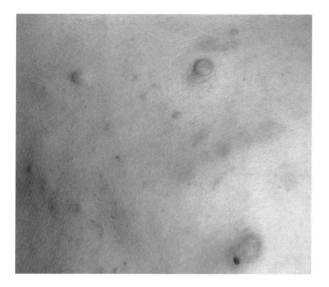

CASE
44

Answers

1 Describe the skin abnormality seen here.
   Multiple flesh-coloured lesions.

2 What is the most likely diagnosis?
   Neurofibromatosis.

3 On which structures do these lesions develop?
   Nerves.

4 The condition is confined to the skin only.
   False.

5 What is the usual pattern of inheritance?
   Autosomal dominant.

6 What other tumours can occur in association with this disorder?
   - *Acoustic neuroma*
   - *Sarcoma.*

7 What other medical disorders are associated with this condition?
   - *Epilepsy*
   - *Phaeochromocytoma.*

CASE
44

CASE 45

Increased pigmentation

This patient has a history of fainting, and of feeling weak and tired.

1 What abnormality is present?

2 What diagnosis would you consider?

3 What is the cause of her syncopal attacks?

4 What investigations would help to confirm the diagnosis?

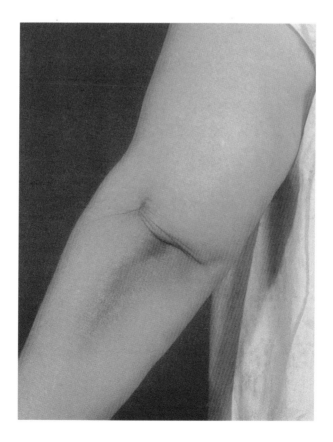

Answers

1 What abnormality is present?

   Pigmentation of the extensor surface of the arm.

2 What diagnosis would you consider?

   Addison's disease.

3 What is the cause of her syncopal attacks?

   Hypotension due to hyponatraemia.

4 What investigations would help to confirm the diagnosis?

   - *Synacthen® test*

   - *Morning cortisol level.*

CASE
45

CASE 46

Tongue and lips

This young man has several lesions on his tongue as well as his lip. He has iron-deficiency anaemia and a history of frequent nosebleeds.

1 What is the nature of the lesions on the lip and tongue?

2 What is the diagnosis?

3 How is this condition most commonly inherited?

   Please tick *one* box:

   Autosomal recessive   ☐

   Autosomal dominant   ☐

   X-linked recessive   ☐

   X-linked dominant   ☐

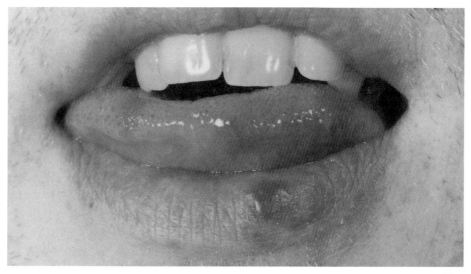

Answers

1 What is the nature of the lesions on the lip and tongue?
   Telangiectatic blood vessels.

2 What is the diagnosis?
   Hereditary telangiectasia/Osler-Weber-Rendu syndrome.

3 How is this condition most commonly inherited?

   Autosomal recessive   ☐

   Autosomal dominant   ☑

   X-linked recessive   ☐

   X-linked dominant   ☐

Clinical signs

CASE
46

CASE 47

The mouth

This young man has recently returned from working in the USA. He has lost weight and has had several episodes of fever and cervical lymphadenopathy.

1 What is the cause of the lesion in the mouth?

2 What conditions may predispose to this disorder?

3 What will you ask this patient about his lifestyle?

His white cell count is normal, but his lymphocyte count is very low and his serum immunoglobulin levels are elevated.

4 What is the most likely diagnosis?

5 What blood tests would confirm this diagnosis?

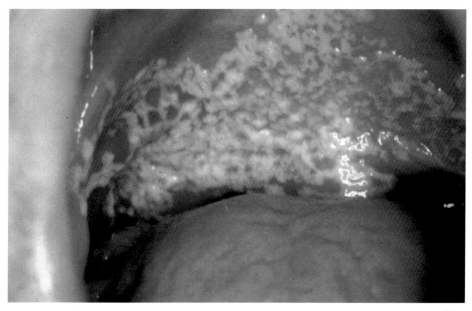

CASE 47

Answers

1 What is the cause of the lesion in the mouth?
  Oral candidiasis.

2 What conditions may predispose to this disorder?
  - *HIV/AIDS*
  - *Underlying malignancy*
  - *Diabetes*
  - *Antibiotic therapy*
  - *Steroid therapy.*

3 What will you ask this patient about his lifestyle?
  Is he in an at-risk group for HIV?

4 What is the most likely diagnosis?
  HIV/AIDS.

5 What blood tests would confirm this diagnosis?
  - *HIV antibody test*
  - *P24 antigen-positive by polymerase chain reaction (PCR) or other HIV antigen test.*

CASE
47

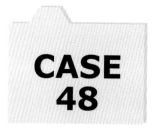

CASE 48

The hands

This woman denies experiencing any pain in her hands at present.

1 What is the diagnosis?

2 What other features would you look for in the upper limbs?

3 What clinical signs indicate disease activity?

4 What blood test can be used to confirm the diagnosis?

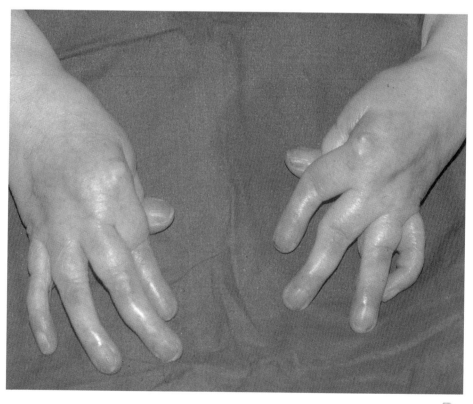

CASE 48

Answers

1 What is the diagnosis?
Rheumatoid arthritis.

2 What other features would you look for in the upper limbs?
- *Rheumatoid nodules*
- *Small-muscle wasting*
- *Ulnar deviation*
- *Subluxation deformities*
- *Z-shaped thumb*
- *Nail fold infarcts*
- *Palmar erythema.*

3 What clinical signs indicate disease activity?
Red, painful, swollen and tender joints.

4 What blood test can be used to confirm the diagnosis?
Rheumatoid factor.

Clinical signs

CASE
48

CASE 49

Nail changes (1)

1 What abnormality is present in this patient?

2 List four possible causes.

3 The patient attends the dermatology clinic. What other nail changes would you expect to find?

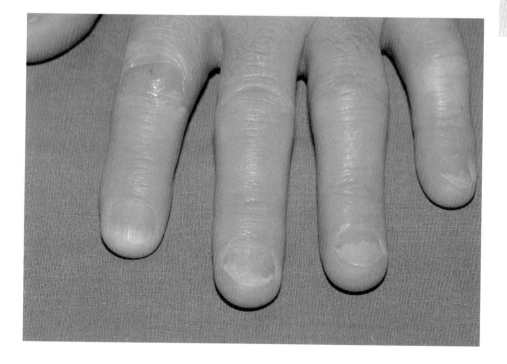

Answers

1 What abnormality is present in this patient?
   Onycholysis.

2 List four possible causes.
   - *Trauma*
   - *Psoriasis*
   - *Thyrotoxicosis*
   - *Drugs.*

3 The patient attends the dermatology clinic. What other changes would you expect to find?
   - *Pitting*
   - *Grease spots*
   - *Nail dystrophy.*

Clinical signs

CASE 49

CASE 50

Nail changes (2)

1 What name is used to describe the nail change seen here?

2 With what deficiency disorder is it associated?

3 What investigations can be used to confirm the diagnosis?

4 This patient developed dysphagia. What complication may have developed to account for this?

5 What investigations could be used to confirm the cause?

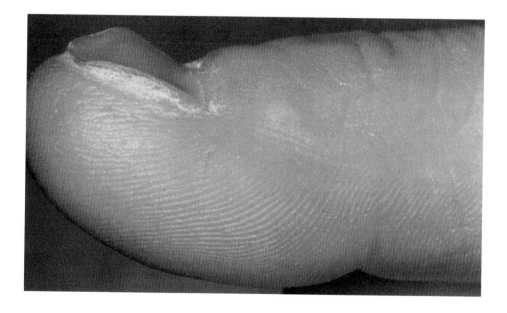

Answers

1 What name is used to describe the nail change seen here?

Koilonychia.

2 With what deficiency disorder is it associated?

Iron deficiency.

3 What investigations can be used to confirm the diagnosis?

- *Serum iron*
- *Total iron-binding capacity (TIBC)*
- *Ferritin.*

4 This patient developed dysphagia. What complication may have developed to account for this?

- *Pharyngeal web/carcinoma*
- *Plummer-Vinson syndrome/Paterson-Brown-Kelly syndrome.*

5 What investigations could be used to confirm the cause?

- *Oesophagogastroduodenoscopy (OGD)*
- *Barium swallow.*

Clinical signs

CASE 50

CASE 51

Nail changes (3)

Look at the photograph of this woman's fingers. She is 63 years old and has complained of a dry cough for over three months.

   1 What abnormality is demonstrated?

   2 What questions would you ask the patient?

   3 What is the first investigation you would order?

   4 What is the most likely diagnosis?

   5 List four other possible causes.

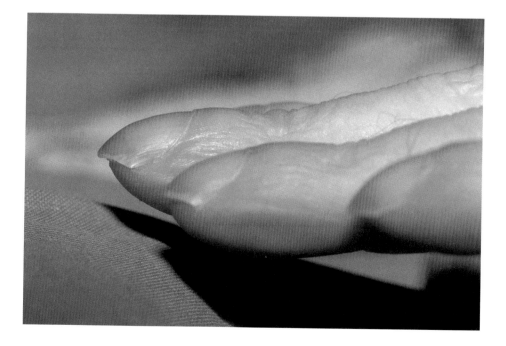

CASE
51

Answers

1 What abnormality is demonstrated?
   Finger clubbing.

2 What questions would you ask the patient?
   - *Smoking status (including passive smoking)*
   - *Haemoptysis*
   - *Hoarseness, chest pain, dyspnoea*
   - *Weight loss*
   - *Occupation, and husband's occupation.*

3 What is the first investigation you would order?
   Chest X-ray.

4 What is the most likely diagnosis?
   Lung neoplasm.

5 List four other possible causes.
   - *Chronic suppurative lung disease*
   - *Arteriovenous malformation*
   - *Bacterial endocarditis*
   - *Chronic diarrhoea*
   - *Cryptogenic fibrosing alveolitis.*

CASE
51

CASE 52

Swollen painful leg

This 34-year-old patient is presenting with a swollen painful leg. He has pyrexia with a temperature of 38.5 °C.

1 What condition does this patient have?

2 What is the commonest causative organism?

3 What name is given to the condition which causes the red linear marks over the knee?

4 What other physical sign would you specifically look for?

5 What treatment is indicated?

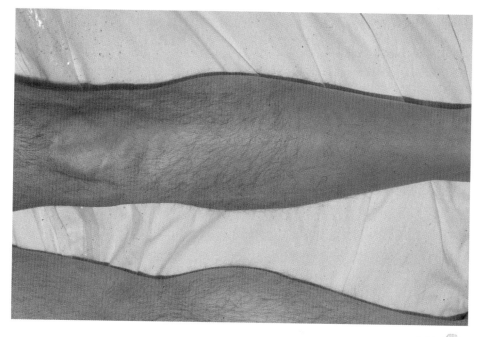

Answers

1 What condition does this patient have?
  Cellulitis.

2 What is the commonest causative organism?
  ß-Haemolytic streptococcus.

3 What name is given to the condition which causes the red linear marks over the knee?
  Ascending lymphangitis.

4 What other physical sign would you specifically look for?
  Tender inguinal lymphadenopathy.

5 What treatment is indicated?
  Penicillin or macrolide antibiotic.

CASE 52

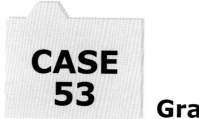

CASE 53

Graves' disease

This woman has Graves' disease.

1 What name is used to describe the clinical appearance of the eye?

2 List the other eye signs that may be present in this condition.

3 What three forms of therapy can be used to treat Graves' disease?

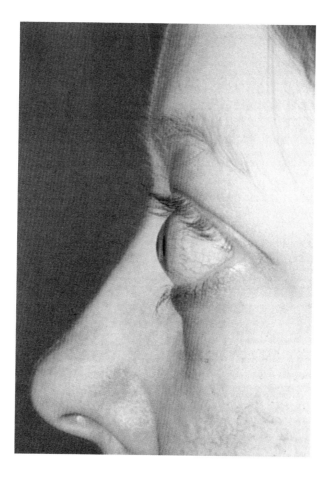

CASE
53

Answers

1 What name is used to describe the clinical appearance of the eye?
   Exophthalmos (proptosis).

2 List the other eye signs that may be present in this condition.
   • *Lid retraction*
   • *Lid lag*
   • *Ophthalmoplegia.*

3 What three forms of therapy can be used to treat Graves' disease?
   • *Surgery*
   • *Antithyroid drug (carbimazole)*
   • *Radioactive iodine.*

CASE 53

CASE 54

Eye sign

This patient was asked to look down.

1 What clinical sign is present?

2 What underlying metabolic disorder causes this clinical sign?

3 List five other symptoms or signs of this condition.

4 What blood test would confirm the diagnosis?

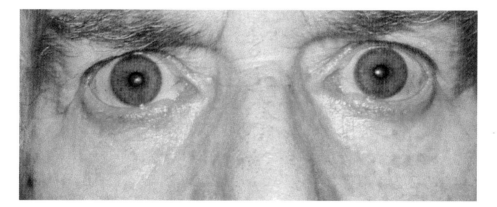

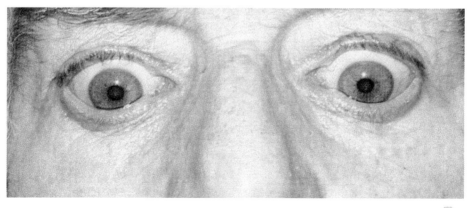

CASE
54

Answers

1 What clinical sign is present?
   Lid lag.

2 What underlying metabolic disorder causes this clinical sign?
   Hyperthyroidism.

3 List five other symptoms or signs of this condition.
   - *Weight loss*
   - *Tremor*
   - *Palpitations*
   - *Heat intolerance*
   - *Anxiety attacks*
   - *Diarrhoea*
   - *Amenorrhoea*
   - *Proptosis*
   - *Ophthalmoplegia*
   - *Goitre.*

4 What blood test would confirm the diagnosis?
   - *Increased serum thyroxine level*
   - *Decreased serum thyroid-stimulating hormone (TSH) level.*

Clinical signs

CASE 54

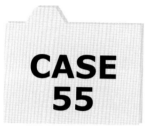

CASE 55

The fundus (1)

1 What abnormalities are present in this photograph of a retina?

2 What is the diagnosis?

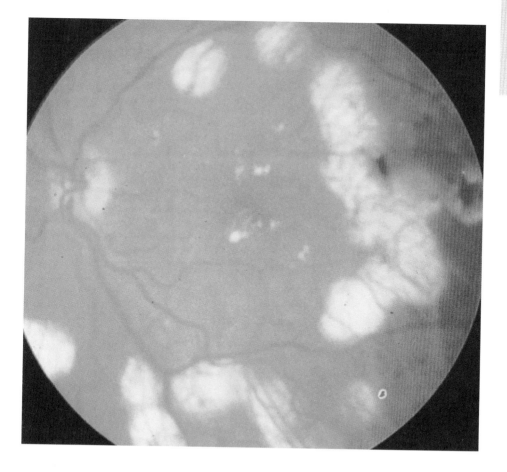

Answers

1 What abnormalities are present in this photograph of a retina?
   - *Hard exudates*
   - *Dot and blot haemorrhages*
   - *Laser photocoagulation scars*
   - *Neovascularisation.*

2 What is the diagnosis?
   Proliferative retinopathy in diabetes.

Clinical signs

CASE
55

CASE 56

The fundus (2)

This is a retinal image from a patient who is completely asymptomatic.

1 What abnormalities are seen on inspection of this retina?

2 What name is given to the white lesion indicated with an arrow?

3 What is the diagnosis?

4 What four classes of drugs are used to treat the condition?

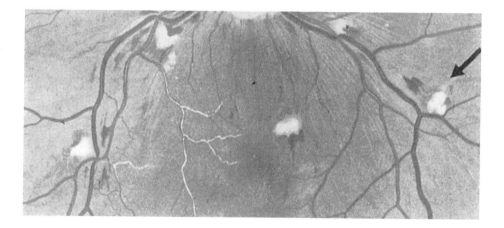

Answers

1 What abnormalities are seen on inspection of this retina?
  - *Flame-shaped haemorrhages*
  - *Cotton-wool spots*
  - *Silver-wiring*
  - *Arteriovenous nipping.*

2 What name is given to the white lesion indicated with an arrow?
  Cotton-wool spots/soft exudates.

3. What is the diagnosis?
  Hypertensive retinopathy.

4. What four classes of drugs are used to treat the condition?
  - *Diuretics*
  - *β-Blockers*
  - *Calcium-channel blocking drugs*
  - *Angiotensin-converting enzyme (ACE) inhibitors or ACE-receptor blockers.*

Clinical signs

CASE 56

CASE 57

The fundus (3)

Clinical signs

A patient presents with progressive loss of power in the right hand and arm, followed by right-sided facial weakness. She describes constant headache, which is felt as a pressure inside the head and is associated with vomiting when the pain is severe. Inspect this photograph of a retina and answer the following questions.

1 What abnormality is present?

2 What cardiovascular signs might be associated with this appearance?

3 What is the most likely underlying cause of this patient's symptoms?

4 A member of the medical staff suggests performing a lumbar puncture to rule out meningitis. What are the risks of performing this procedure?

5 What drug therapy could you use in this patient to give temporary relief of symptoms?

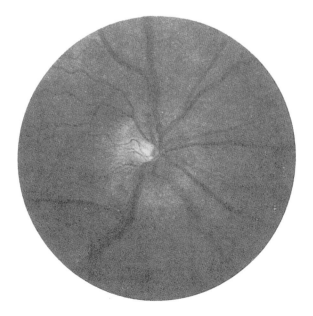

CASE 57

Answers

1 What abnormality is present?
   Blurring of the optic nerve head – papilloedema.

2 What cardiovascular signs might be associated with this appearance?
   - *Bradycardia*
   - *Hypertension.*

3 What is the most likely underlying cause of this patient's symptoms?
   Raised intracranial pressure due to a tumour.

4 A member of the medical staff suggests performing a lumbar puncture to rule out meningitis. What are the risks of performing this procedure?
   Coning of the brain leading to sudden death.

5 What drug therapy could you use in this patient to give temporary relief of symptoms?
   Dexamethasone.

Clinical signs

CASE
57

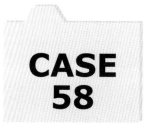

CASE 58

The fundus (4)

A 72-year-old patient presents with poor vision in the left eye and is unable to read even large newsprint. This is the appearance of the fundus.

1 What abnormality is seen on inspection of the left fundus?

2 What name is given to this condition?

3 List three causes.

4 The patient has a past history of muscle pain and stiffness affecting the shoulder girdle and upper arms. What blood test would you request and what result would you expect?

5 What name is given to the disorder that is causing muscle pain and stiffness?

6 What treatment is indicated to prevent further visual impairment?

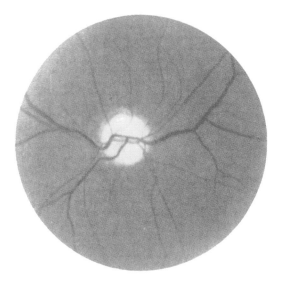

Answers

1 What abnormality is seen on inspection of the left fundus?
  Pale optic nerve head.

2 What name is given to this condition?
  Optic atrophy.

3 List three causes.
  - *Giant-cell arteritis*
  - *Embolus*
  - *Multiple sclerosis.*

4 The patient has a past history of muscle pain and stiffness affecting the shoulder girdle and upper arms. What blood test would you request and what result would you expect?
  Erythrocyte sedimentation rate (ESR) > 100 mm in the first hour.

5 What name is given to the disorder that is causing muscle pain and stiffness?
  Polymyalgia rheumatica.

6 What treatment is indicated to prevent further visual impairment?
  High-dose steroids.

Clinical signs

CASE
58

Clinical examination

Marking overall score for clinical examination stations

0	Unsatisfactory	Major deficiencies in clinical skills
		No systematic approach
		Little or no concern for the patient
		Missed diagnosis, even with prompting
1	Below average	Minor deficiencies in clinical skills
		Not experienced in performing examination
		Reached diagnosis with help/prompting
2	Satisfactory	Competent clinical skills
		Systematic examination
		Reached diagnosis unaided
		Sympathy with patient
3	Excellent	Highly competent clinical skills
		Systematic and professional examination
		Diagnosis and differential diagnosis reached
		Suggested other findings
		Patient-centred examination

Clinical examination

CASE 59

The pulse

Instructions for student

This patient has an abnormal pulse. Examine their pulse and inform the examiner of your findings.

Instructions for examiner

The student has been asked to examine the pulse only. The patient has one of the following conditions:

- atrial fibrillation
- plateau pulse (aortic stenosis)
- collapsing pulse (aortic incompetence).

Marking schedule

Introduction to the patient.

Obtained consent for examination.

Explanation of the examination to be performed.

Palpated both radial arteries.

Rate.

Rhythm.

Volume.

Character.

Vessel wall.

Diagnosis.

Causes.

Knowledge of other associated clinical signs.

Able to name one investigation that would confirm the diagnosis.

Overall score: **0   1   2   3**   **(please circle one)**

CASE 59

CASE 60

Auscultation of the heart

Instructions for student

Use your stethoscope to auscultate this patient's heart. Inform the examiner of your findings.

Instructions for examiner

The student has been instructed to auscultate the precordium of this patient, who has one of these cardiac conditions:

- mitral stenosis
- mitral incompetence
- aortic stenosis
- aortic incompetence
- aortic stenosis and incompetence
- aortic and mitral valve disease
- atrial septal defect
- ventricular septal defect.

Marking schedule

Introduction to the patient.

Obtained consent for examination.

Explanation of the examination to be performed.

Located apex beat.

Auscultated all areas of precordium systematically.

Positioned patient to maximise likelihood of hearing murmurs.

Used respiratory phases to maximise likelihood of hearing murmurs.

Systematic reporting of findings (from first heart sound, systole, second heart sound, diastole).

Correct findings.

Able to list common causes.

Knowledge of possible associated clinical signs.

Could list investigations to confirm the diagnosis.

Overall score: 0   1   2   3   **(please circle one)**

**CASE
60**

CASE 61

Jugular venous system

Instructions for student

Examine the jugular venous system of this patient and inform the examiner of your findings.

CASE 61

Instructions for examiner

The student has been asked to examine the neck veins of this patient, who has one of the following conditions:

- right ventricular failure
- superior vena caval obstruction
- constrictive pericarditis
- pericardial effusion.

Marking schedule

Introduction to the patient.

Obtained consent for examination.

Explanation of the examination to be performed.

Position of patient at 45 degrees.

Identification of internal and external jugular veins.

Recognition of findings:

- degree of elevation/upper level
- presence/absence of waveforms
- amplitude of waveforms.

Hepatojugular reflux:

- ask about abdominal tenderness
- explain procedure
- tell patient to breathe normally
- establish correct findings.

Correct diagnosis.

Overall score: 0   1   2   3   **(please circle one)**

CASE
61

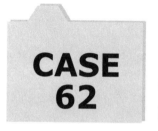

CASE 62

Blood pressure recording

Instructions for student

This patient complains of feeling faint when they stand up from either a sitting or a lying position. Using the equipment provided, perform the relevant examination to determine the cause.

Clinical examination

CASE
62

Instructions for examiner

You are a patient with postural hypotension. The student has been informed that you feel faint on standing up from either a sitting or a lying position.

The student must measure your blood pressure when you are lying down and then when you are standing.

Marking schedule

Introduction to the patient.

Obtained consent.

Explanation of the procedure.

Blood pressure recorded from patient lying down.

Technique:

- position of cuff
- location of brachial pulse
- systolic pressure by palpation obtained first
- three measurements obtained by auscultation
- accuracy of measurements
- fully deflates cuff between recordings.

Blood pressure recorded from patient while standing.

Patient advised to lie down if they feel faint.

Knowledge of definition of postural hypotension (fall of systolic pressure by > 10 mmHg).

Overall performance: 0   1   2   3   **(please circle one)**

Clinical examination

CASE 62

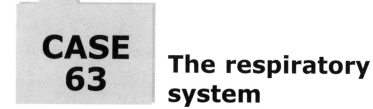

CASE 63

The respiratory system

Instructions for student

Examine this patient's respiratory system. Marks will be given for the following:

1 Examination technique:

   - expansion
   - percussion
   - auscultation.

2 Interpretation of findings.

Instructions for examiner

The student has been asked to examine the chest expansion in this patient, and to percuss and auscultate the patient's chest. The patient has one of the following conditions:

- a pleural effusion
- chronic obstructive lung disease
- asthma
- pulmonary fibrosis
- bronchiectasis.

Marking schedule

Introduction.

Obtained consent for examination.

Examination of chest expansion.

Technique for percussing chest.

Systematic auscultation of the lungs.

Interpretation of clinical findings.

Diagnosis obtained.

Differential diagnosis.

Overall score:　　　　**0**　　**1**　　**2**　　**3**　　　**(please circle one)**

Clinical examination

CASE
63

CASE 64

The abdomen

Instructions for student

Please perform a physical examination of this patient's abdomen. You are not required to perform a rectal examination.

Clinical examination

Instructions for examiner

The student has been instructed to perform an examination of the abdomen but not a rectal examination. The patient has one of the following abnormalities of the abdomen:

- liver enlargement
- liver and spleen enlargement
- splenomegaly
- abdominal distension due to ascites
- polycystic kidney disease
- ectopic kidney (in renal transplant patient).

Marking schedule

Introduction to the patient.

Obtained consent for examination.

Explanation of the examination to be performed.

Asked about abdominal tenderness.

Inspection carried out.

Light palpation.

Deep palpation (all nine regions).

Palpation for liver.

Percussion for liver.

Palpation for spleen.

Percussion for spleen.

Bimanual palpation for kidneys.

Percussion for ascites.

Test for shifting dullness.

Test for fluid thrill.

Auscultation for bowel sounds.

Washed hands after examination.

Overall score:　　　　**0**　　　**1**　　　**2**　　　**3**　　　**(please circle one)**

CASE
64

Clinical examination

CASE 65

The joints

Instructions for student

This patient is complaining of joint pains. Please examine their hands to determine the nature of the underlying disorder.

Instructions for examiner

The student has been asked to examine the hands of this patient who may have:

- rheumatoid arthritis
- psoriatic arthritis
- osteoarthritis.

Marking schedule

Introduction to the patient.

Obtained consent for examination.

Asked about pain or tenderness.

General inspection.

Recognised abnormalities.

Looked for associated signs in hands.

Tested range of movements.

Tested functional movements:

- opening buttons
- lifting cup/glass
- opening bottle, etc.

Looked for associated signs in the rest of the body (eg rheumatoid nodules – rheumatoid arthritis, skin rash – psoriasis).

Overall score: 0 1 2 3 **(please circle one)**

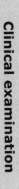

Clinical examination

CASE
65

CASE 66

The fundus

Instructions for student

Using an ophthalmoscope, please inspect the fundus of this patient (a mannequin) and describe any abnormalities that are present.

Clinical examination

Instructions for examiner

The student has been instructed to examine this fundus which has classic features of one of the following conditions:

- hypertensive retinopathy
- diabetic retinopathy with or without laser scars
- optic atrophy
- papilloedema.

Marking schedule

Introduction to the patient.

Obtained consent for examination.

Explained procedure.

Enquired about vision and use of glasses.

Inspected both eyes.

Recognised and described abnormalities.

Accurate diagnosis.

Knowledge of commonest underlying causes.

Technique using ophthalmoscope.

Overall score: **0**   **1**   **2**   **3**   **(please circle one)**

CASE
66

CASE 67

General inspection

Instructions for student

You are required to report to the examiner any abnormalities you can observe on general inspection of this patient.

Clinical examination

Instructions for examiner

The student has been instructed that after general inspection of this patient they should report any abnormalities they have observed. The patient may have:

- hyperthyroidism (Graves' disease)
- hypothyroidism
- acromegaly
- Cushing's syndrome
- Addison's disease
- Marfan's syndrome
- chronic liver disease
- haemochromatosis
- scleroderma/CREST syndrome
- systemic lupus erythematosus.

Marking schedule

Introduction.

Obtained consent for examination.

Clinical findings (give one mark for each).

Graves' disease:

- exophthalmos
- lid retraction
- lid lag
- goitre
- characteristics of gland
- sweating
- tachycardia
- thin
- fine tremor.

Hypothyroidism:

- overweight
- dry coarse hair
- loss of outer third of eyebrows
- pale
- goitre
- characteristics of gland
- hung-up reflexes

CASE
67

- cold
- bradycardia.

Acromegaly:

- large hands
- large mandible
- frontal bossing
- coarse features
- bitemporal hemianopia
- large heel pad
- large tongue.

Cushing's syndrome:

- moon face
- buffalo hump
- central obesity
- peripheral wasting
- hirsutism
- myopathy
- striae.

Addison's disease:

- extensor pigmentation
- buccal pigmentation
- pigmented palmar creases
- hypotension
- pigmented scars.

Marfan's syndrome:

- tall
- long arms
- arachnodactyly
- dislocation of the lens
- aortic or mitral murmurs
- scars from previous chest drains.

Chronic liver disease:

- jaundice
- spider naevi
- fetor hepaticus
- thin skin
- gynaecomastia

Clinical examination

CASE
67

- loss of male secondary sexual characteristics
- testicular atrophy
- constructional apraxia
- ascites
- peripheral oedema
- asterixis
- telangiectasia
- caput medusae
- finger clubbing
- palmar erythema.

Haemochromatosis:

- hyperpigmentation
- features of liver disease (see above).

Scleroderma/CREST syndrome:

- calcinosis
- Raynaud's phenomenon
- sclerodactyly
- telangiectasia
- trophic lesions on digits.

Systemic lupus erythematosus:

- discoid or lupus rash
- vasculitic rash
- non-deforming arthritis
- mouth ulceration
- alopecia
- Raynaud's phenomenon.

Overall score: 0   1   2   3   **(please circle one)**

CASE
67

CASE 68

Muscle power, tone and reflexes

Instructions for student

Examine the muscle power, tone and reflexes in the upper and lower limbs of this patient and report your findings to the examiner.

Instructions for examiner

The student has been instructed to examine the muscle power, tone and reflexes in the upper and lower limbs of this patient. The patient may have:

- left/right hemiparesis
- motor neurone disease
- spastic paraparesis
- Parkinson's disease/parkinsonism.

Marking schedule

Introduction to the patient.

Obtained consent for examination.

Explanation of the examination.

Examination of all muscle groups.

Marks for technique:

- power
- tone
- reflexes.

Abnormalities detected.

Diagnosis achieved.

Knowledge of grades of power.

Knowledge of types of abnormal tone.

Ability to differentiate between upper and lower motor neurone lesions.

Overall score: 0   1   2   3   **(please circle one)**

CASE
68

CASE 69

Sensation

Instructions for student

This patient has had problems with loss of sensation in their arms/legs. Please perform a physical examination to determine the nature of the sensory loss and the most likely cause.

Instructions for examiner

The student has been asked to examine sensation in this patient's arms/legs. They should report the type of sensory loss and the most common underlying cause. The patient may have:

1 Peripheral neuropathy due to:
   - diabetes mellitus
   - vitamin B_{12} deficiency
   - alcohol.
2 Mononeuropathy due to:
   - carpal tunnel syndrome
   - ulnar nerve compression.
3 Sensory nerve root compression.
4 Spinal cord demyelination – multiple sclerosis.

Marking schedule

Introduction to the patient.

Obtained consent for the examination.

Explanation of the examination procedure.

Comparison of both sides of the body.

Tested all sensory modalities:

- pain (pinprick)
- temperature
- touch
- vibration
- proprioception.

Correct identification of sensory deficits.

Correct identification of type of sensory loss.

Knowledge of commonest causes.

Overall score: 0   1   2   3   (please circle one)

CASE
69

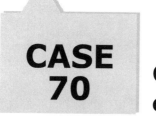

CASE 70

Cranial nerve examination

Instructions for student

Please demonstrate to the examiner how you would examine all of the cranial nerves on this simulated patient.

CASE
70

Instructions for examiner

The student must demonstrate how they would perform an assessment of the cranial nerves within five minutes.

Marking schedule

Introduction to the patient.

Obtained consent for the examination.

Explanation of the examination procedure.

Cranial nerves:

- I – used smelling salts, tested nostrils individually
- II – used Snellen chart correctly plus newsprint
- III, IV and VI – tested full range of eye movements
- V – tested sensory and motor functions
- VII – tested muscle groups above and below the eyes
- VIII – tested hearing and confirmed air greater than bone conduction
- IX, X – observed palatal movement
- XI – tested trapezius and/or sternomastoids
- XII – asked patient to protrude the tongue.

Overall score: **0   1   2   3**   **(please circle one)**

Clinical examination

CASE
70

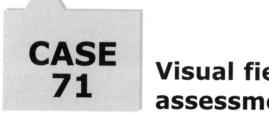

CASE 71

Visual field assessment

Instructions for student

This patient is complaining of headache and visual disturbance. Test the patient's visual fields.

Instructions for examiner

You are a patient with symptoms of headache and a visual field defect. The student has been instructed to test your visual fields. They should perform visual fields assessment by confrontation. Please simulate one of the following visual field defects:

- left/right homonymous hemianopia
- bitemporal hemianopia
- left/right supraquadrantic defect.

Marking schedule

Introduction to the patient.

Consent obtained for the examination.

Technique for performing the confrontation test.

Established visual field defect.

Knowledge of possible cause of the defect.

Overall score: **0   1   2   3   (please circle one)**

**CASE
71**

CASE 72

Cerebellar function

Instructions for student

This patient has fallen over while washing her face. She feels unsteady while walking and have had numerous falls. Perform a neurological examination to determine the underlying cause.

Clinical examination

CASE
72

Instructions for examiner

You have symptoms of unsteadiness and a history of numerous falls, especially on closing your eyes – for example, during face washing.

Please simulate all of the following symptoms of cerebellar disease:

- positive Romberg's sign
- wide-spaced stamping gait
- left/right-sided intention tremor, past-pointing, dysdiadochokinesia
- scanning speech.

Marking schedule

Introduction to the patient.

Consent obtained for the examination.

Assessment of gait.

Assessment of speech.

Romberg's sign.

Finger–nose test.

Heel–shin test.

Test for dysdiadochokinesia.

Detection of abnormalities.

Diagnosis of cerebellar disease.

Overall score: **0**   **1**   **2**   **3**   **(please circle one)**

CASE 72

CASE 73

Mental state

Instructions for student

This patient has been confused and exhibiting abnormal behaviour. Please perform an assessment of the patient's mental state.

CASE
73

Instructions for examiner

The simulated patient has been trained to display features of a confusional state. The student has been instructed to assess the patient's mental state. Then ask the student:

1 To name one cause of a chronic confusional state

2 To classify the causes of acute confusional states.

Marking schedule

Introduction to the patient.

Consent obtained for the examination.

Assessment of orientation:

- time
- person
- place.

Assessment of short-term memory.

Assessment of attention and calculation (eg serial sevens).

Assessment of language skills:

- name objects
- repeat nonsense phrase
- perform a written instruction
- write down a dictated sentence
- perform a verbal instruction.

Assessment of visuospatial skills (eg copy a drawing of a geometric pattern).

Causes of chronic confusion – one of:

- senile dementia
- cerebral ischaemia
- multi-cerebral infarcts.

Classification of acute confusional states – one mark for each mentioned from:

- alcohol or alcohol withdrawal
- drugs
- major organ failure
- neurological disorders (epilepsy or encephalitis)
- raised intracranial pressure
- metabolic/endocrine disorders (includes electrolyte, fluid or acid–base imbalance)
- head injury/trauma
- hypoxia or hypercapnia.

Overall score: 0   1   2   3   **(please circle one)**

CASE
73

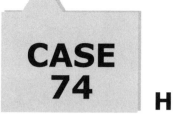

CASE 74

Hearing

Instructions for student

This patient has a hearing defect. Please assess their hearing and, using the equipment provided, determine the nature of the hearing deficit.

Instructions for examiner

You are a patient with a hearing deficit. The student must assess your hearing and, using the tuning fork, determine the nature of your deafness.

Please simulate either:

- conductive deafness in the left or right ear, or
- nerve deafness in the left or right ear.

Marking schedule

Introduction to the patient.

Consent obtained for the examination.

Explanation of the examination procedure.

Assessment of hearing acuity:

- each ear tested separately
- determination of severity of hearing loss
- standing behind the patient while testing.

Use of tuning fork:

- Weber's test
- Rinne's test.

Correct diagnosis of the hearing deficit.

Overall score: **0**   **1**   **2**   **3**   **(please circle one)**

CASE 74

CASE 75

The joints

Instructions for student

This patient has joint pains. Please perform an assessment of the musculoskeletal system to determine the underlying disorder and assess its severity.

Instructions for examiner

This student has been instructed to examine the musculoskeletal system of the patient with joint pain at this station, and to determine the underlying cause and assess the severity of the disorder.

The patient has one of the following:

- rheumatoid arthritis
- osteoarthritis of one large joint
- ankylosing spondylitis
- systemic lupus erythematosus
- psoriatic arthropathy
- gout.

Marking schedule

Introduction to the patient.

Consent obtained for the examination.

Inspection – observed all abnormalities.

Palpation:

- for tenderness
- for change in temperature
- for swelling.

Tested range of movement of affected joints:

- passive movement
- range of active movement.

Functional tests (eg for hands – holding cup, opening buttons, opening jars; for lower limbs – walking).

Tests for ankylosing spondylitis – assessment of spinal flexion, extension and lateral flexion.

Overall score: 0   1   2   3   **(please circle one)**

CASE
75

X-ray

CASE 76

Sudden chest pain and dyspnoea

This X-ray was taken from a 24-year-old man who suddenly developed chest pain and breathlessness while playing football.

1 What abnormalities are visible?

2 Name three underlying disorders that could cause this abnormality.

3 If the patient became cyanosed and distressed due to shortness of breath, what complication could have developed?

4 What clinical signs would confirm that this had occurred?

5 What action should be taken?

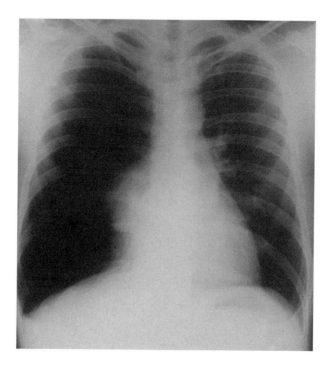

Answers

1 What abnormalities are visible?
   - *No lung markings on right side*
   - *Lung edge visible at hilum.*

2 Name three underlying disorders that could cause this abnormality.
   - *Marfan's syndrome*
   - *Emphysema*
   - *Lung abscess*
   - *Tuberculosis*
   - *Trauma.*

3 If the patient became cyanosed and distressed due to shortness of breath, what complication could have developed?
   Tension pneumothorax.

4 What clinical signs would confirm that this had occurred?
   Deviation of the trachea to the opposite side.

5 What action should be taken?
   Insertion of cannula to release tension.

X-ray

CASE
76

CASE 77

Increasing dyspnoea

This X-ray was taken from a patient with severe shortness of breath that had developed over a two-hour period.

1 List four abnormalities which can be clearly seen.

2 What is the most likely diagnosis?

3 List two possible causes of the sudden onset of symptoms.

4 What drugs are used in the emergency management of this condition?

X-ray

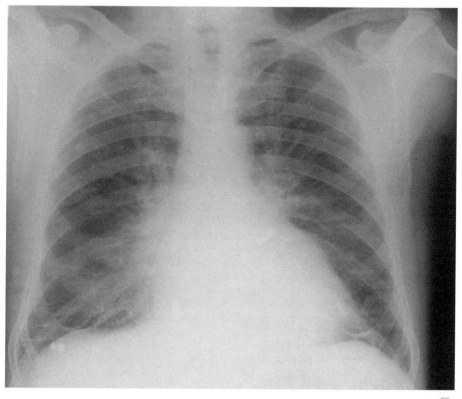

CASE
77

Answers

1 List four abnormalities which can be clearly seen.
- *Cardiomegaly*
- *Prominent upper lobe veins*
- *Kerley B lines*
- *Peribronchial shadowing.*

2 What is the most likely diagnosis?
Acute left ventricular failure or pulmonary oedema.

3 List two possible causes of the sudden onset of symptoms.
- *Myocardial infarction*
- *Cardiac arrhythmia*
- *Acute valvular dysfunction*
- *Acute septal rupture.*

4 What drugs are used in the emergency management of this condition?
- *Intravenous diuretic*
- *Diamorphine*
- *Oxygen*
- *Aminophylline.*

X-ray

CASE
77

CASE 78

Recurrent chest infections and weight loss

This patient has had four hospital admissions in the past six months for chest infection. Over the past four months she has lost 2 kg in body weight, associated with loss of appetite.

1 What abnormality is present on this chest X-ray?

2 List two possible causes.

3 The patient has features of Cushing's syndrome. What is the most likely cause?

4 What treatment would cure the Cushing's syndrome?

X-ray

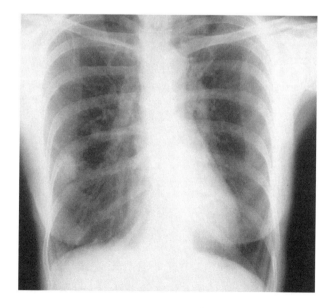

Answers

1 What abnormality is present on this chest X-ray?
   Rounded opacity at periphery of right lung.

2 List two possible causes.
   - *Primary lung cancer*
   - *Secondary lung tumour*
   - *Rheumatoid nodule*
   - *Round pneumonia*
   - *Arteriovenous malformation.*

3 The patient has features of Cushing's syndrome.
   What is the most likely cause?
   Adrenocorticotropic hormone (ACTH)-secreting small-cell carcinoma of the lung.

4 What treatment would cure the Cushing's syndrome?
   Resection of the lung tumour.

X-ray

CASE
78

CASE 79

Fever, cough and herpes labialis

This 18-year-old patient has a five-day history of fever, cough and general malaise. He is not short of breath at rest, and he has a herpes simplex lesion on his upper lip.

1 Describe the abnormalities that are evident on this patient's chest X-ray.

2 What is the diagnosis?

3 What is the most likely causative agent?

4 What other investigation should be performed?

5 What treatment would be most appropriate?

X-ray

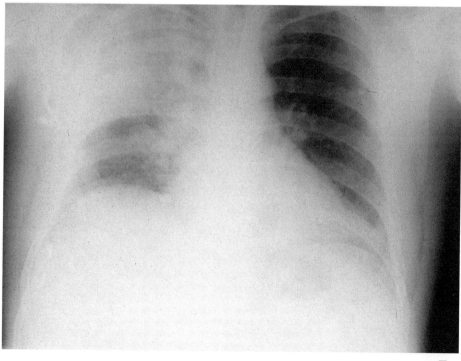

CASE
79

Answers

1 Describe the abnormalities that are evident on this patient's chest X-ray.
  Consolidation of the right mid-zone and upper lobe.

2 *What is the diagnosis?*
  Lobar pneumonia.

3 What is the most likely causative agent?
  Streptococcus pneumoniae.

4 What other investigation should be performed?
  - *Total and differential white cell count*
  - *Sputum culture*
  - *Blood culture*
  - *C-reactive protein.*

5 What treatment would be most appropriate?
  - *Penicillin antibiotic*
  - *Antipyretic.*

X-ray

CASE
79

CASE 80

Recurrent pleuritic pains

This woman has had five episodes of sudden sharp chest pains, sometimes associated with shortness of breath. The pain lasts for 30–60 seconds and then resolves. It can affect both the left and right sides and is usually felt in the back. The patient has a past history of three spontaneous miscarriages and hypertension.

1 What abnormalities are present on the patient's chest X-ray?

2 What is the most likely cause of these abnormalities?

3 What other investigations would be useful to confirm the diagnosis?

4 What is the significance of the patient's past obstetric history?

5 What treatment should be given for this most recent episode?

6 For how long should treatment be continued?

X-ray

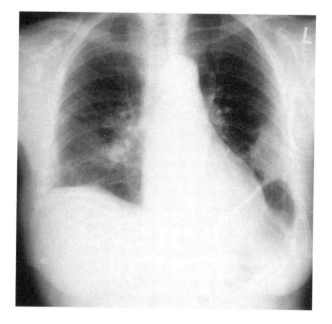

CASE
80

Answers

1 What abnormalities are present on the patient's chest X-ray?
- *Raised hemidiaphragms*
- *Wedge-shaped area of consolidation on the left side.*

2 What is the most likely cause of these abnormalities?
  Recurrent pulmonary emboli.

3 What other investigations would be useful to confirm the diagnosis?
- *Spiral CT scan*
- *Pulmonary arteriography*
- *Ventilation-perfusion scan*
- *D-dimer test.*

4 What is the significance of the patient's past obstetric history?
- *Possible antiphospholipid antibody syndrome*
- *Protein S or protein C deficiency.*

5 What treatment should be given for this most recent episode?
  Low molecular weight heparin and then warfarin.

6 For how long should treatment be continued?
  Lifelong.

X-ray

CASE
80

CASE 81

Fever and haemoptysis

This elderly patient has been unwell for two weeks with fevers, cough and shortness of breath. He has recently coughed up some bloodstained sputum.

1 What abnormalities can be seen on the chest X-ray?

2 What is the diagnosis?

3 What is the most likely causative agent?

4 What drug treatment would be indicated?

5 What investigation would you request to confirm the diagnosis and the underlying cause?

6 What other form of management may be necessary?

X-ray

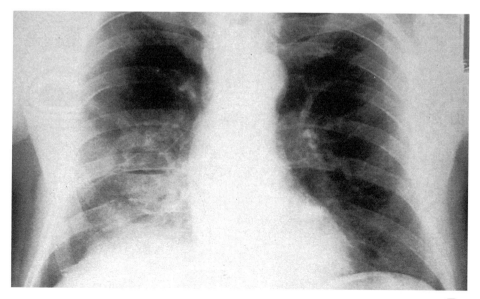

CASE 81

Answers

1 What abnormalities can be seen on the chest X-ray?
   Consolidation of the right mid zone with air/fluid level.

2 What is the diagnosis?
   Lung abscess secondary to bronchopneumonia.

3 What is the most likely causative agent?
   Staphylococcus.

4 What drug treatment would be indicated?
   Flucloxacillin.

5 What investigation would you request to confirm the diagnosis and the underlying cause?
   - *Sputum culture*
   - *Blood culture during episode of fever*
   - *CT scan of the chest*
   - *Bronchoscopy.*

6 What other form of management may be necessary?
   Percutaneous drainage.

X-ray

CASE
81

CASE 82

Dysphagia

This patient has a three-month history of difficulty in swallowing solids. He occasionally regurgitates undigested food.

1 What type of X-ray is shown?

2 What abnormalities are shown?

3 What is the most likely diagnosis?

4 List three further causes of oesophageal narrowing.

5 What confirmatory investigation could be performed?

6 What further investigation(s) would be required before surgery is undertaken?

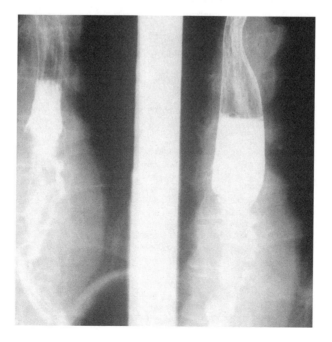

Answers

1 What type of X-ray is shown?
   Barium swallow.

2 What abnormalities are shown?
   - *Dilated oesophagus*
   - *Irregular narrowing at lower end of the oesophagus*
   - *Fluid level.*

3 What is the most likely diagnosis?
   Carcinoma of the oesophagus.

4 List three further causes of oesophageal narrowing.
   - *Achalasia*
   - *Peptic stricture*
   - *Ingestion of corrosive liquid*
   - *Radiotherapy*
   - *Long-term placement of a nasogastric tube.*

5 What confirmatory investigation could be performed?
   Endoscopy of upper gastrointestinal tract with biopsy.

6 What further investigation(s) would be required before surgery is
   undertaken?
   - *CT scan*
   - *Endoscopic ultrasound scan to stage the tumour accurately.*

X-ray

CASE
82

CASE 83

Change in bowel habit

This 78-year-old man has a three-month history of constipation.

1 What type of X-ray is shown?

2 Describe what is shown in this contrast picture.

3 What is the most likely diagnosis?

4 How could this diagnosis be confirmed?

5 What gastrointestinal conditions can predispose to this disorder?

6 What other investigations should be carried out?

7 What treatment is indicated?

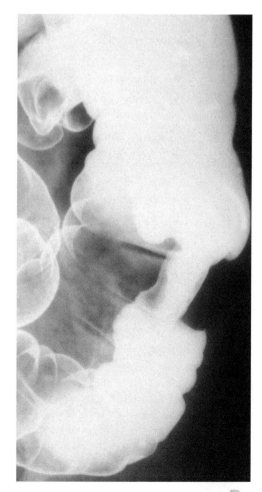

X-ray

Answers

1 What type of X-ray is shown?
  Barium enema.

2 Describe what is shown in this contrast picture.
  Large bowel with an area of narrowing. The narrowed region has irregular edges and an 'apple core' appearance.

3 What is the most likely diagnosis?
  Carcinoma of the colon.

4 How could this diagnosis be confirmed?
  By sigmoidoscopy or colonoscopy with biopsy.

5 What gastrointestinal conditions can predispose to this disorder?
  - *Colonic polyps (adenomas)*
  - *Inflammatory bowel disease*
  - *Familial polyposis syndrome.*

6 What other investigations should be carried out?
  - *Full blood picture – for anaemia*
  - *Liver function tests*
  - *Ultrasound scan of the abdomen*
  - *Faecal occult blood test.*

7 What treatment is indicated?
  Surgical resection.

X-ray

CASE
83

CASE 84

Crampy abdominal pain

This X-ray was taken of a 22-year-old law student with a history of episodes of crampy central abdominal pain associated with frequent bowel motions and occasional diarrhoea. He has lost 3 kg in body weight over the past year, and also complains of painful gums which occasionally bleed.

1 What type of X-ray is shown?

2 Describe any abnormalities which you can identify.

3 What is the most likely diagnosis?

4 What non-gastrointestinal features can be associated with this disorder?

5 What blood tests will be abnormal?

6 What drug treatments are used for this condition?

X-ray

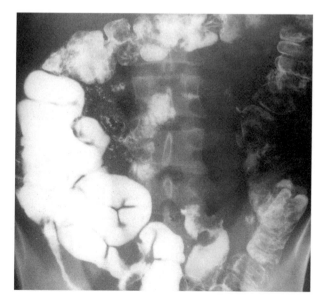

CASE 84

Answers

1 What type of X-ray is shown?
   Small bowel barium contrast study.

2 Describe any abnormalities which you can identify.
   * *Areas of narrowing of the lumen*
   * *Thickened bowel wall*
   * *Abnormal communications – fistulae.*

3 What is the most likely diagnosis?
   Crohn's disease.

4 What non-gastrointestinal features can be associated with this disorder?
   * *Uveitis/scleritis*
   * *Sacroiliitis*
   * *Erythema nodosum*
   * *Gallstones*
   * *Renal stones.*

5 What blood tests will be abnormal?
   * *Full blood picture – may show anaemia*
   * *Erythrocyte sedimentation rate – elevated*
   * *C-reactive protein – elevated*
   * *Biochemistry – may show malabsorption.*

6 What drug treatments are used for this condition?
   * *Steroids*
   * *Sulfasalazine*
   * *Azathioprine*
   * *Infliximab.*

X-ray

CASE
84

CASE 85

Gradually increasing dyspnoea

This patient has an eight-month history of gradually increasing shortness of breath.

1 Describe the X-ray shown below as if you were the radiologist preparing the report.

2 What is the diagnosis?

3 What clinical signs are characteristically found on examination?

4 What further procedure is necessary to try to determine the cause?

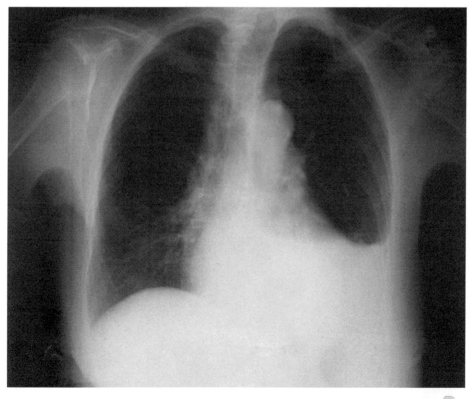

Answers

1 Describe the X-ray as if you were the radiologist preparing the report.
- *Posterior–anterior X-ray*
- *Identify patient and date taken*
- *Rotation*
- *Inspiratory effort*
- *Penetration of film*
- *Obvious – pleural effusion on left side*
- *Pleural disease*
- *Bony skeleton*
- *Diagnosis.*

2 What is the diagnosis?
Left-sided pleural effusion.

3 What clinical signs are characteristically found on examination?
- *Reduced expansion on the affected side*
- *Possible deviation of trachea to the opposite side*
- *Stony-dull percussion note*
- *Absent or reduced breath sounds*
- *Reduced vocal resonance and fremitis*
- *Signs at the fluid level – bronchial breath sounds, increased vocal resonance, whispering pectoriloquy, aegophony.*

4 What further procedure is necessary to try to determine the cause?
Pleural aspiration for estimation of protein content, bacteriology and cytology.

X-ray

CASE
85

Data interpretation

CASE 86

Full blood picture (1)

A 65-year-old woman presents to a hospital outpatient clinic with a history of tiredness, breathlessness and lack of energy. Her full blood picture result is as follows:

	Observed value	Normal range
Haemoglobin	6.8 g/dl	12–17
Packed cell volume (PCV)	0.47	0.36–0.54
Mean corpuscular volume	112 fl	90–100
Mean corpuscular haemoglobin	34.5 pg	27–32
Mean corpuscular haemoglobin concentration	37.8 g/dl	32–36

1 What descriptive terms are used to describe these findings?

2 List two possible causes in this patient.

3 What investigations would determine the cause?

4 What would be the typical features on bone marrow examination?

Data interpretation

CASE
86

Answers

1 What descriptive terms are used to describe these findings?
   Macrocytic hyperchromic anaemia.

2 List two possible causes in this patient.
   - *Vitamin B_{12} deficiency in the diet*
   - *Folate deficiency in the diet*
   - *Pernicious anaemia*
   - *Malabsorption.*

3 What investigations would determine the cause?
   - *Serum vitamin B_{12} and folate*
   - *Schilling test*
   - *Anti-parietal cell or anti-intrinsic factor antibodies*
   - *Malabsorption screen*
   - *Bone marrow examination.*

4 What would be the typical features on bone marrow examination?
   Megaloblastic bone marrow.

CASE
86

CASE 87

Full blood picture (2)

This is a full blood picture of a 38-year-old woman with a three-month history of tiredness and lack of energy which is getting progressively worse.

	Observed value	Normal range
Haemoglobin	8.2 g/dl	11–15
White cell count	7.4 x 10^9/l	4–11
Mean corpuscular haemoglobin	5.4 pg	27–32
Mean corpuscular haemoglobin concentration	29 g/dl	32–36
Mean corpuscular volume	74 fl	90–100
Platelets	250 x 10^9/l	150–400

1 How would you describe this blood picture?

2 What is the commonest cause?

3 What blood tests will confirm the diagnosis?

4 List three possible causes.

5 What drug therapy is best used?

6 What should the duration of this therapy be after the haemoglobin value reaches the normal range? (please circle the correct answer)

3 days   3 weeks   3 months   1 year

Data interpretation

CASE
87

Answers

1 How would you describe this blood picture?
   Microcytic hypochromic anaemia.

2 What is the commonest cause?
   Iron deficiency.

3 What blood tests will confirm the diagnosis?
   - *Serum iron*
   - *Percentage saturation*
   - *Total iron-binding capacity*
   - *Serum ferritin.*

4 List three possible causes.
   - *Dietary deficiency*
   - *Malabsorption*
   - *Blood loss – menstrual, gastrointestinal tract or urinary tract.*

5 What form of drug therapy is best used?
   Ferrous salts administered orally.

6 What should the duration of this therapy be after the haemoglobin value
   reaches the normal range?
   3 months.

CASE
87

Data interpretation

CASE 88

Full blood picture and biochemical profile

A 42-year-old woman is admitted with pain in her lumbar spine, tiredness and lack of energy. On examination she is pale and has tenderness over L2 to L4. The investigation results are as follows:

	Observed value	Normal range
Haemoglobin	9.2 g/dl	12–17
White cell count	2.5×10^9/l	4–11
Platelets	58×10^9/l	150–400
Erythrocyte sedimentation rate	124 mm/first hour	< 20
Sodium	140 mmol/l	135–145
Potassium	4.2 mmol/l	3.5–4.5
Urea	6.1 mmol/l	3.3–8.8
Total protein	110 g/l	55–80
Albumin	42 g/l	35–50
Calcium	3.1 mmol/l	2.2–2.6
IgG	24.1 g/l	4–12
IgM	1.5 g/l	1.2–4.0
IgA	1.4 g/l	0.5–2.5

1 What is the most likely diagnosis?

2 What abnormalities might be seen on X-ray of the bony skeleton?

3 What urine test would help to confirm the diagnosis?

4 What abnormality would be seen on bone marrow biopsy?

5 What name is given to the changes in the full blood picture?

6 What treatment is given for the primary disease?

7 What inflammatory joint condition can complicate this disease or arise after treatment has started?

Data interpretation

CASE
88

Answers

1   What is the most likely diagnosis?
    Multiple myeloma.

2   What abnormalities might be seen on X-ray of the bony skeleton?
    Lytic lesions, generalised oeteoporosis or pathological fractures.

3   What urine test would help to confirm the diagnosis?
    Urinary Bence Jones proteins.

4   What abnormality would be seen on bone marrow biopsy?
    Increased number of plasma cells.

5   What name is given to the changes in full blood picture?
    Pancytopenia.

6   What treatment is given for the primary disease?
    Melphalan – cytotoxic drug therapy.

7   What inflammatory joint condition can complicate this disease or arise after treatment has started?
    Gout.

CASE
88

Data interpretation

CASE 89

Biochemical profile and liver function tests

An 18-year-old girl has a two-week history of anorexia, nausea and vomiting. She has lost 2.4 kg in weight. The biochemical results of liver function tests and electrolytes are shown:

	Observed value	Normal range
Sodium	143 mmol/l	135–145
Potassium	3.5 mmol/l	3.5–4.5
Chloride	102 mmol/l	98–108
Urea	4.1 mmol/l	3.3–8.8
Albumin	41 g/l	35–50
Bilirubin	26 μmol/l	3.3–18
γ-Glutamyl transferase	58 U/l	0–30
Alkaline phosphatase	114 U/l	30–120
Aspartate aminotransferase	231 U/l	0–40
Alanine aminotransferase	320 U/l	0–40

1 What condition would these results suggest?

2 What further investigations are indicated to determine the cause?

3 What will you specifically ask the patient about?

4 What investigation results would indicate an infective cause?

Data interpretation

CASE
89

Answers

1 What condition would these results suggest?
   Hepatocellular jaundice.

2 What further investigations are indicated to determine the cause?
   Viral screening tests for viral hepatitis and cytomegalovirus.

3 What will you specifically ask the patient about?
   - *Contact with anyone jaundiced*
   - *Foreign travel*
   - *Blood transfusion*
   - *Sexual contact*
   - *Intravenous drug use*
   - *Alcohol intake*
   - *Exposure to drugs/chemicals/anaesthetic agents.*

4 What investigation results would indicate an infective cause?
   - *Raised white cell count*
   - *Viral-specific immunoglobulins*
   - *Viral antigen detection.*

Data interpretation

CASE 89

CASE 90

Liver function tests

A 60-year-old woman presents with weight loss and abdominal pain. Her liver function tests are as follows:

	Observed value	Normal range
Alanine aminotransferase	41 U/l	0–30
Alkaline phosphatase	199 U/l	30–120
Aspartate aminotransferase	34 U/l	0–40
Bilirubin	121 μmol/l	< 17
γ-Glutamyl transferase (GGT)	89 U/l	0–30

1 What condition would these results suggest?

2 Give three possible causes.

3 List three further investigations.

4 If the gallbladder is easily felt on abdominal examination, which cause is less likely?

5 The auto antibody screening tests show a high level of antimitochondrial antibody. What condition would you consider?

Data interpretation

CASE 90

Answers

1 What condition would these results suggest?
   Obstructive jaundice.

2 Give three possible causes.
   - *Gallstones*
   - *Carcinoma of the head of pancreas*
   - *External pressure on the biliary system*
   - *Stricture or narrowing of the bile ducts.*

3 List three further investigations.
   - *Ultrasound scan of the abdomen*
   - *CT scan*
   - *ERCP.*

4 If the gallbladder is easily felt on abdominal examination, which cause is less likely?
   Gallstones.

5 The autoantibody screening tests show a high level of antimitochondrial antibody. What condition would you consider?
   Primary biliary cirrhosis.

Data interpretation

CASE 90

CASE 91

Renal profile tests

Miss Alison Jones is a young woman with swelling of both lower legs and around both eyes. She feels generally unwell and has slight shortness of breath on exertion. Investigation results are as follows:

	Observed value	Normal range
Sodium	148 mmol/l	135–145
Potassium	5.0 mmol/l	3.3–4.5
Chloride	110 mmol/l	98–108
Urea	19.5 μmol/l	3.3–8.8
Creatinine	200 μmol/l	40–110
Albumin	26 g/l	35–50

Urine analysis:

- Protein   +++
- Blood   ++
- Glucose   Nil

Urine volume in 24 hours: 250 ml

Urine microscopy:

- Red cells   ++
- Pus cells   +++
- Casts present

Urine creatinine: 40 mmol/l

1 What condition is this patient suffering from?
2 How is this condition classified?
3 If the patient has had a normal blood pressure and there is no evidence of urinary retention, what type of the condition is most likely to be present?
4 What is the patient's creatinine clearance/glomerular filtration rate?
5 What total volume of fluid intake will you permit in the next 24 hours?
6 What dietary regime will you request?
7 What oral treatment can be given to prevent any further increase in the serum potassium level?
8 If the serum potassium level rises to 6 mmol/l, what treatment can be given to rapidly reduce the potassium level?
9 If this fails to control the rising potassium level, what treatment would be necessary?

Data interpretation

CASE 91

Answers

1 What condition is this patient suffering from?
   Acute renal failure.

2 How is this condition classified?
   - *Pre-renal*
   - *Renal*
   - *Post-renal.*

3 If the patient has had a normal blood pressure and there is no evidence of urinary retention, what type of the condition is most likely to be present?
   Renal.

4 What is the patient's creatinine clearance/glomerular filtration rate?
   40 ml/minute.

5 What total volume of fluid intake will you permit in the next 24 hours?
   750 ml.

6 What dietary regime will you request?
   - *Low-protein*
   - *Low-potassium*
   - *High-calorie.*

7 What oral treatment can be given to prevent any further increase in the serum potassium level?
   Ion-exchange resin (eg Calcium Resonium®).

8 If the serum potassium level rises to 6 mmol/l, what treatment can be given to rapidly reduce the potassium level?
   - *50 ml of 50% dextrose intravenously*
   - *10 units of insulin intramuscularly.*

9 If this fails to control the rising potassium level, what treatment would be necessary?
   Dialysis.

CASE 91

CASE 92

Full blood picture, biochemistry and renal function tests

A 42-year-old woman with a 20-year history of insulin-dependent diabetes mellitus is admitted complaining of tiredness, muscle weakness, bone pains and nausea, which have developed over the past six months. Her full blood picture, routine biochemical tests and urine tests are shown. After careful inspection of these results, please answer the questions overleaf.

Full blood picture

	Observed value	Normal range
Haemoglobin (Hb)	7.4 g/dl	12–17
Mean corpuscular volume	92 fl	90–100
Mean corpuscular Hb	30 pg	27–32
Mean corpuscular Hb concentration	34 g/dl	32–36
White cell count	6.3×10^9/l	4–11
Platelets	248×10^9/l	150–400

Routine biochemistry

	Observed value	Normal range
Sodium	142 mmol/l	135–145
Potassium	5.0 mmol/l	3.5–4.5
Chloride	102 mmol/l	98–108
Urea	24.3 mmol/l	3.3–8.8
Creatinine	500 μmol/l	40–110
Albumin	28 g/l	35–50

Data interpretation

CASE 92

Blood glucose	12.3 mmol/l	3.3–6.6
Hb A$_{1C}$	10.5%	< 7
Calcium	1.9 mmol/l	2.2–2.6
Phosphate	1.5 mmol/l	0.8–1.6
Alkaline phosphatase	110 U/l	35–120

Urine tests

Urine volume in 24 hours: 1000 ml

Urine creatinine: 22.5 mmol/l

1 What abnormalities are present in the biochemical analysis?

2 What is the most likely cause of the urea and creatinine results?

3 How would you describe the full blood picture?

4 What is the underlying disease?

5 What is this patient's approximate glomerular filtration rate (creatinine clearance)?

6 What is the normal glomerular filtration rate?

7 What dietary regime would you advise?

8 What treatment can be used to treat the patient's anaemia?

9 What is the cause of her low serum calcium level?

10 How can this calcium disorder be corrected?

11 Despite therapy, this woman develops progressive renal failure. What long-term management should be considered?

CASE
92

Answers

1 What abnormalities are present in the biochemical analysis?
- *Increased urea levels*
- *Increased creatinine levels*
- *Poorly controlled diabetes*
- *Hypoalbuminaemia*
- *Hyperkalaemia.*

2 What is the most likely cause of the urea and creatinine results?
   Diabetic nephropathy.

3 How would you describe the full blood picture?
   Normochromic normocytic anaemia.

4 What is the underlying disease?
   Chronic renal failure.

5 What is this patient's approximate glomerular filtration rate (creatinine clearance)?
   45 ml/minute.

6 What is the normal glomerular filtration rate?
   110–120 ml/minute.

7 What dietary regime would you advise?
   Low-protein, low-potassium diet.

8 What treatment can be used to treat the patient's anaemia?
   Erythropoietin injections.

9 What is the cause of her low serum calcium level?
   Impaired metabolism of vitamin D.

10 How can this calcium disorder be corrected?
   By giving 1-α-hydroxycholecalciferol.

Data interpretation

CASE
92

11 Despite therapy, this woman develops progressive renal failure. What long-term management should be considered?

- *Dialysis*
- *Renal transplantation.*

Data interpretation

CASE
92

CASE 93

Bone profile

An 80-year-old woman is referred to the clinic with pain in her left hip region. There are no abnormal physical findings, and in particular she has full range of movement of the left hip joint. A bone profile is requested and this shows the following:

	Observed value	Normal range
Albumin	38 g/l	30–50
Calcium	2.5 mmol/l	2.2–2.6
Phosphate	0.92 mmol/l	0.8–1.6
Alkaline phosphatase	305 U/l	35–120
Total protein	68 g/l	55–80

1 What diagnosis would you consider?

2 What X-rays will you request?

3 What treatment is used for this condition?

Data interpretation

CASE
93

Answers

1 What diagnosis would you consider?
    Paget's disease of bone.

2 What X-rays will you request?
    • *Both hip joints*
    • *Pelvis.*

3 What treatment is used for this condition?
    • *Analgesics*
    • *Bisphosphonates.*

CASE
93

CASE 94

Cerebrospinal fluid tests

A 22-year-old university student is admitted with a history of fever, headache and a skin rash. On examination he has neck stiffness and a positive Kernig's sign. There is a widespread petechial rash. A CT scan of the brain shows no evidence of raised intracranial pressure or haemorrhage. A lumbar puncture is performed. Cerebrospinal fluid (CSF) is obtained by lumbar puncture and shows the following:

	Observed	Normal
CSF appearance	Cloudy	Clear
CSF pressure	25 cm H_2O	10–20
White cell count	600 neutrophils/ml	< 5
Protein content	2 g/l	< 0.4
Glucose CSF/blood ratio	35%	> 70%

1 What is the cause of this patient's headache?

2 What is the most likely aetiological agent?

3 What risk factors would you ask about?

4 What additional investigations should be performed on the CSF sample?

5 What treatment is indicated? Please name a class of drug and route of administration.

6 What can be done to prevent other students from contracting this disorder?

Data interpretation

224 Essential Skills Practice for OSCEs in Medicine

Answers

1 What is the cause of this patient's headache?
   Meningitis.

2 What is the most likely aetiological agent?
   Meningococcal organism (Neisseria meningitidis).

3 What risk factors would you ask about?
   - *Living in student block accommodation*
   - *Other students affected*
   - *Recent sore throat.*

4 What additional investigations should be performed on the CSF sample?
   - *Direct microscopy*
   - *Culture.*

5 What treatment is indicated? Please name a class of drug and route of administration.
   Benzylpenicillin antibiotic administered intravenously.

6 What can be done to prevent other students from contracting this disorder?
   - *Antibiotics given to close contacts*
   - *Vaccine for other students in the institution.*

Data interpretation

CASE
94

CASE 95

Pleural fluid biochemistry

A 68-year-old retired shipyard worker is admitted with increasing shortness of breath. Clinical examination and chest X-ray show a moderately large right-sided pleural effusion with no signs of pulmonary oedema. Some pleural fluid is aspirated and biochemical analysis shows the following:

Colour	Straw-coloured
Protein content	42 g/l
Lactic dehydrogenase	325 U/l

1 What type of pleural effusion is present?

2 Why is it important to measure the lactic dehydrogenase activity as well as the protein content?

3 List the main possible causes of this patient's pleural effusion.

4 About exposure to which occupational hazard will you specifically enquire?

5 What other history will you specifically ask about?

6 What additional investigations should be performed on the pleural fluid?

Data interpretation

CASE
95

Answers

1 What type of pleural effusion is present?

  Exudate.

2 Why is it important to measure the lactic dehydrogenase activity as well as the protein content?

  Patients with hypoproteinaemia will not show a high protein content in exudates, but the lactic dehydrogenase activity will be more than 200 U/l.

3 List the main possible causes of this patient's pleural effusion.

- *Bronchogenic carcinoma*
- *Mesothelioma*
- *Asbestosis.*

4 About exposure to which occupational hazard will you specifically enquire?

  Asbestos.

5 What other history will you specifically ask about?

  Cigarette smoking.

6 What additional investigations should be performed on the pleural fluid?

- *Bacteriological culture*
- *Cytology for malignant cells*
- *Glucose assay*
- *pH*
- *Staining and culture for tuberculosis.*

CASE
95

CASE 96

ECG: chest pain

1 What abnormalities are present on this ECG taken from a 49-year-old patient admitted with a history of chest pain for one hour?

2 What is the diagnosis?

3 What treatment should be given?

4 What complications can occur within the next two hours?

5 The patient develops acute shortness of breath, and on examination a loud systolic murmur is audible. What complication has developed?

6 What will the chest X-ray show?

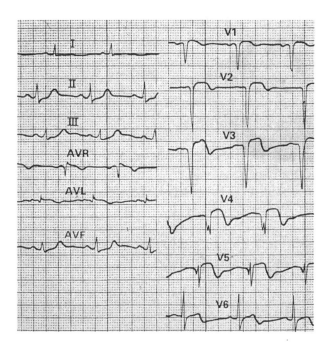

CASE
96

Answers

1 What abnormalities are present on this ECG taken from a 49-year-old patient admitted with a history of chest pain for one hour?

ST elevation and T-wave inversion on anterior leads (I, AVL and V leads).

2 What is the diagnosis?

Anterior myocardial infarction.

3 What treatment should be given?

- *Aspirin therapy*
- *Morphine or diamorphine for pain relief*
- *Anti-emetic*
- *Oxygen by inhalation*
- *Thrombolysis if there are no contraindications.*

4 What complications can occur within the next two hours?

- *Asystolic arrest*
- *Ventricular tachycardia*
- *Ventricular fibrillation*
- *Acute pulmonary oedema*
- *Septal or ventricular wall rupture*
- *Papillary muscle dysfunction.*

5 The patient develops acute shortness of breath, and on examination a loud systolic murmur is audible. What complication has developed?

Acute papillary muscle dysfunction or acute mitral incompetence.

6 What will the chest X-ray show?

Evidence of pulmonary oedema and cardiomegaly.

Data interpretation

CASE
96

CASE 97

ECG: sudden collapse

This ECG was taken from a patient who suddenly collapsed in a surgical unit seven days after abdominal surgery. On examination the patient was found to be short of breath and cyanosed, with a blood pressure of 90/50 mmHg.

1 What abnormalities are present on the standard leads of the ECG?

2 What is the cardiac rate?

3 What abnormalities are seen on inspection of the chest leads?

4 What is the diagnosis?

5 What abnormality would you specifically listen for on auscultation of the heart?

6 What blood test may help to confirm the diagnosis?

7 What other tests can be used to confirm the diagnosis?

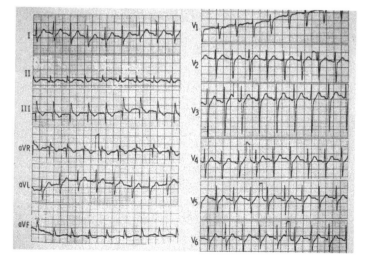

CASE
97

Data interpretation

Answers

1 What abnormalities are present on the standard leads of the ECG?
- *S1 (deep S wave on lead I)*
- *Q3 (Q wave on lead III)*
- *T-wave inversion on lead III.*

2 What is the cardiac rate?
130 beats/minute.

3 What abnormalities are seen on inspection of the chest leads?
QRS widening on V1 to V4.

4 What is the diagnosis?
Pulmonary embolism.

5 What abnormality would you specifically listen for on auscultation of the heart?
A loud pulmonary component of the second heart sound.

6 What blood test may help to confirm the diagnosis?
Elevated D-dimers.

7 What other tests can be used to confirm the diagnosis?
- *Ventilation-perfusion scan of the lungs*
- *Spiral CT scan of the chest*
- *Pulmonary angiography.*

Data interpretation

CASE
97

CASE 98

ECG: elderly patient

This is the ECG of a patient with ischaemic heart disease.

1 What abnormalities are present on this ECG?

2 What underlying conditions can cause this type of ECG?

3 What may precipitate this in a susceptible patient?

4 What are the principal aims of therapy for this condition?

5 If the condition cannot be reversed, what additional drug treatment should be initiated?

6 If this additional treatment is not given, what complications can arise?

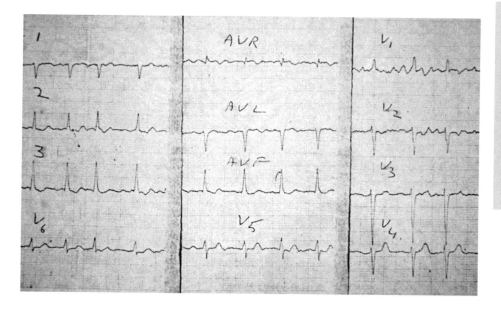

CASE
98

Answers

1 What abnormalities are present on this ECG?
- *ECG shows irregularly irregular rhythm*
- *Absence of P waves*
- *Diagnosis of atrial fibrillation.*

2 What underlying conditions can cause this type of ECG?
- *Ischaemic heart disease*
- *Mitral valve disease·*
- *Thyrotoxicosis*
- *After myocardial infarction*
- *Alcoholic cardiomyopathy.*

3 What may precipitate this in a susceptible patient?
- *Infection*
- *Electrolyte disturbance*
- *Pulmonary embolism*
- *Excess caffeine*
- *Excess alcohol.*

4 What are the principal aims of therapy for this condition?
- *Treat any underlying cause*
- *Revert to sinus rhythm if possible*
- *Maintain apical rate at < 100/minute.*

5 If the condition cannot be reversed, what additional drug treatment should be initiated?
   Warfarin anticoagulation.

6 If this additional treatment is not given, what complications can arise?
- *Left atrial thrombus*
- *Embolic events*
- *Transient ischaemic attack/stroke.*

CASE 98

Data interpretation

CASE 99

ECG: stabbing chest pains

This ECG was recorded from a 26-year-old man who has chest pain, fever, shortness of breath and a raised white blood cell count.

1 What abnormalities are present?

2 What is the differential diagnosis?

3 The elevated white cell count is due to lymphocytosis. What is the most likely cause?

4 What other conditions can cause this disorder?

5 What complication can develop as a result of this condition?

6 What are the characteristic clinical signs which would indicate that this complication has occurred?

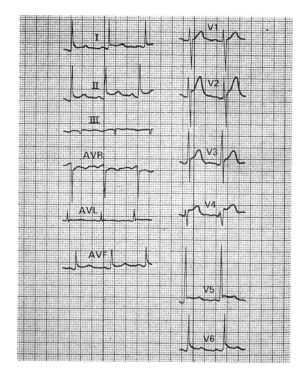

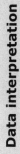

Data interpretation

CASE 99

Answers

1 What abnormalities are present?

   ST elevation (concave upwards) in most leads.

2 What is the differential diagnosis?
   - *Pericarditis*
   - *Myocardial infarction*
   - *Prinzmetal's variant angina.*

3 The elevated white cell count is due to lymphocytosis. What is the most likely cause?

   Viral pericarditis.

4 What other conditions can cause this disorder?
   - *Myocardial infarction*
   - *Uraemia*
   - *Connective tissue disease (eg systemic lupus erythematosus, rheumatoid arthritis)*
   - *After cardiac surgery*
   - *Trauma*
   - *Sarcoidosis*
   - *Bacterial infection.*

5 What complication can develop as a result of this condition?
   - *Pericardial effusion*
   - *Constrictive pericarditis.*

6 What are the characteristic clinical signs which would indicate that this complication has occurred?
   - *Muffled heart sounds*
   - *Raised jugular venous pressure (JVP)*
   - *Reduced amplitude of JVP waves*
   - *Pulsus paradoxus.*

CASE 99

CASE 100

ECG: muscle weakness

This ECG was taken from a patient who had muscle weakness. There was a past history of hypertension and acute renal impairment.

1 What abnormalities are present?

2 What is the diagnosis?

3 Name one underlying cause.

4 What blood test would you perform as an emergency?

5 If you found an abnormally high result (> 6.0 mmol/l), outline what treatment you would administer.

6 If this treatment failed to correct the abnormality, what treatment would you suggest?

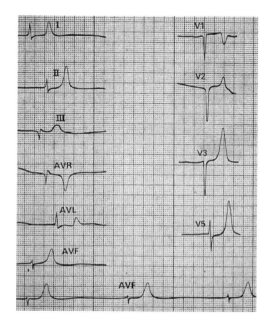

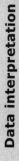

CASE
100

Answers

1 What abnormalities are present?
- *Tall, peaked T waves*
- *Reduced R waves*
- *Widening QRS complexes*
- *Prolonged PR interval.*

2 What is the diagnosis?
Hyperkalaemia.

3 Name one underlying cause.
- *Renal failure*
- *Drug-induced.*

4 What blood test would you perform as an emergency?
Serum potassium.

5 If you found an abnormally high result (> 6.0 mmol/l), outline what treatment you would administer.
50 ml of 50% dextrose plus 10 units of insulin.

6 If this treatment failed to correct the abnormality, what treatment would you suggest?
Peritoneal dialysis or haemodialysis.

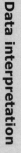

Data interpretation

CASE
100

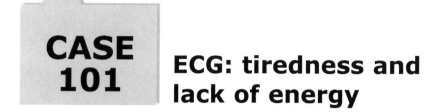

CASE 101

ECG: tiredness and lack of energy

This ECG recording was taken from a 57-year-old patient with a history of weight gain and cold intolerance. She feels tired and lethargic.

1 What abnormalities are present?

2 What is the most likely cause of the ECG appearance in this case?

3 What other conditions can cause a similar ECG appearance?

4 What blood tests would be abnormal?

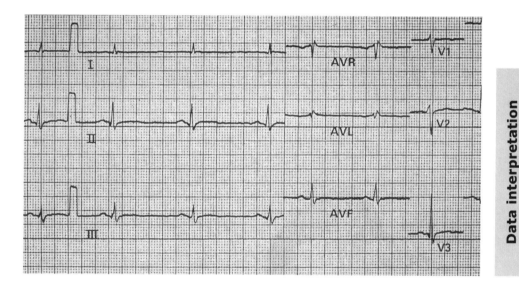

Data interpretation

Answers

1 What abnormalities are present?
- *Bradycardia*
- *Low-voltage QRS complexes.*

2 What is the most likely cause of the ECG appearance in this case?
   Hypothyroidism.

3 What other conditions can cause a similar ECG appearance?
- *Drugs (eg ß-blockers)*
- *Hypothermia*
- *Obesity.*

4 What blood tests would be abnormal?
- *Reduced thyroxine*
- *Increased thyroid-stimulating hormone*
- *Increased creatine kinase*
- *Increased cholesterol.*

CASE
101

CASE 102

ECG: transient weakness

This ECG was taken from a patient admitted with transient weakness of the left arm and leg and left facial weakness. She recovered power within six hours.

1 What abnormalities are evident?

2 What is the likely cause of the ECG changes?

3 What name is given to the neurological condition?

4 How may the ECG changes be responsible for the neurological event?

5 Which blood tests would be useful to confirm the cardiac abnormality?

6 In approximately what percentage of cases do patients present with a neurological event secondary to a cardiac disorder?
   (please circle the correct answer)

   1%   5%   15%   25%

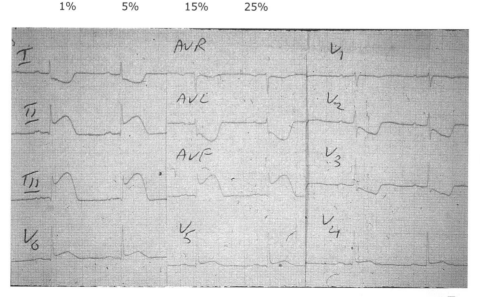

Data interpretation

Answers

1   What abnormalities are evident?
   - *ST elevation and T-wave inversion II, III and AVF in leads with reciprocal changes in anterior leads.*

2   What is the likely cause of the ECG changes?
   Inferior myocardial infarction.

3   What name is given to the neurological condition?
   Transient ischaemic attack.

4   How may the ECG changes be responsible for the neurological event?
   - *Hypotensive episode or arrhythmia after infarction*
   - *Embolism from a mural or left ventricular thrombus.*

5   Which blood tests would be useful to confirm the cardiac abnormality?
   - *Troponin elevation*
   - *Cardiac enzymes.*

6   In approximately what percentage of cases do patients present with a neurological event secondary to a cardiac disorder?
   5%.

Data interpretation

CASE
102

CASE 103

ECG: syncopal attacks

This ECG was recorded from a patient with a history of syncopal attacks (sudden loss of consciousness lasting for 30–60 seconds followed by full recovery).

1 Describe any abnormality which can be seen.

2 What is the mechanism whereby this results in syncope?

3 What are the commonest causes of this cardiac abnormality?

4 In which region of the heart does this abnormality arise?

5 What treatment is used and why?

6 Name one drug that can be given intravenously to treat this disorder in the acute phase.

7 What other form of treatment can be used?

8 What else can be done to prevent repeated attacks of collapse in this patient?

Data interpretation

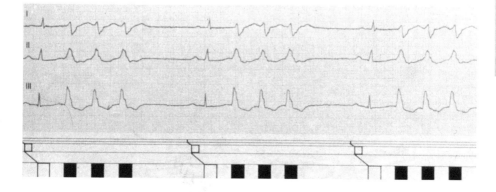

CASE 103

While in hospital, the patient had a further episode of collapse during which the blood pressure was unrecordable and the ECG shown below was recorded.

9 What disorder is shown?

10 What treatment would you initiate?

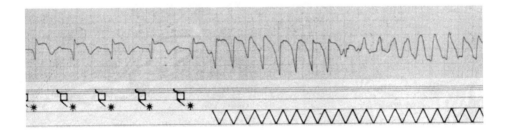

CASE 103

Answers

1 Describe any abnormality which can be seen.
   Ventricular ectopics/ventricular tachycardia.

2 What is the mechanism whereby this results in syncope?
   Transient hypotension.

3 What are the commonest causes of this cardiac abnormality?
   • *After myocardial infarction*

   • *Ischaemic heart disease*

   • *Cardiomyopathy.*

4 In which region of the heart does this abnormality arise?
   The left or right ventricle.

5 What treatment is used and why?
   *Anti-arrhythmic drugs are used to reduce the risk of sustained
      tachycardia or ventricular fibrillation.*

6 Name one drug that can be given intravenously to treat this disorder in the
   acute phase.
   • *Lidocaine (lignocaine) 50 mg over 2 minutes, and then 2
      mg/minute by infusion*

   • *Amiodarone 300 mg over 5–15 minutes.*

7 What other form of treatment can be used?
   DC conversion.

8 What else can be done to prevent repeated attacks of collapse in this
   patient?
   Implanted defibrillator.

Data interpretation

CASE
103

9 While in hospital, the patient had a further episode of collapse during which the blood pressure was unrecordable and a second ECG was recorded.
What disorder is shown in this ECG?
  Ventricular fibrillation.

10 What treatment would you initiate?
  Basic life support until defibrillation can be carried out.

CASE
103

CASE 104

ECG: after exercise stress test

This is a 12-lead ECG taken from a patient immediately after an exercise stress test.

1 What is the heart rate?

2 What abnormalities are present?

3 What is the diagnosis?

4 Which regions of the heart are affected?

5 What risk factors would you ask about or determine?

6 What further investigations would you feel are indicated?

7 List three classes of drugs which could be used to treat this condition, and give the mechanism of action of each.

8 What other form of therapy might be considered?

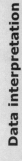

Data interpretation

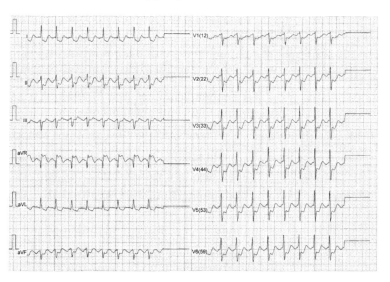

CASE
104

Answers

1 What is the heart rate?
    130 beats/minute.

2 What abnormalities are present?
    Widespread ST depression and all leads.

3 What is the diagnosis?
    Ischaemic heart disease.

4 Which regions of the heart are affected?
    Anterior and inferior walls of the left ventricle.

5 What risk factors would you ask about or determine?
- *Body weight*
- *History of diabetes, hypertension or smoking*
- *Family history*
- *Cholesterol level.*

6 What further investigations would you feel are indicated?
- *Echocardiography*
- *Coronary arteriography.*

7 List three classes of drugs which could be used to treat this condition, and give the mechanism of action of each.
- *Nitrates – vasodilation*
- *β-Blockers – reduced heart rate and reduced force of contraction*
- *Calcium-channel blockers – reduced peripheral resistance.*

8 What other form of therapy might be considered?
- *Angioplasty and stent*
- *Coronary artery bypass grafting.*

Data interpretation

CASE 104

CASE 105

ECG: chronic renal disease

This ECG was recorded from a 48-year-old woman who has a ten-year history of chronic pyelonephritis.

1 What abnormalities can be seen on examination of this resting ECG?

2 What cardiac abnormality is present?

3 List the two commonest causes.

4 What might you expect to hear on auscultation of the heart?

5 What other clinical examination is indicated that is directly relevant to the ECG features?

6 What classes of drugs are used to treat this disorder?

7 Apart from renal disease, list four other causes of this disorder.

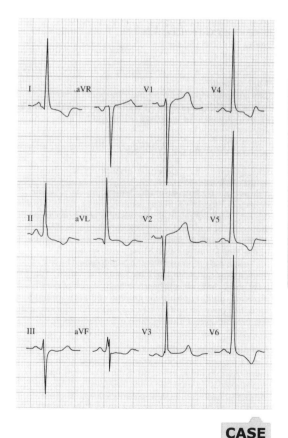

CASE
105

Answers

1 What abnormalities can be seen on examination of this resting ECG?
  - *Large R waves and deep S waves in V leads*
  - *T waves inversionin leads I, II, AVL and V4 to V6.*

2 What cardiac abnormality is present?
  Left ventricular hypertrophy.

3 List the two commonest causes.
  - *Hypertension*
  - *Aortic valve disease.*

4 What might you expect to hear on auscultation of the heart?
  - *Aortic systolic murmur*
  - *Fourth heart sound.*

5 What other clinical examination is indicated that is directly relevant to the ECG features?
  - *Blood pressure recording*
  - *Examination of the retina – hypertensive changes.*

6 What classes of drugs are used to treat this disorder?
  - *Diuretics*
  - *ß-Blockers*
  - *Calcium antagonists*
  - *ACE inhibitors*
  - *ACE receptor-blocking drugs.*

Data interpretation

**CASE
105**

7 Apart from renal disease, list four other causes of this disorder.

- *Essential hypertension*

- *Pregnancy/pre-eclampsia*

- *Renal artery stenosis*

- *Cushing's syndrome*

- *Conn's syndrome*

- *Phaeochromocytoma*

- *Acromegaly*

- *Drugs (oral contraceptive pill, hormone replacement therapy, steroids).*

Data interpretation

CASE
105

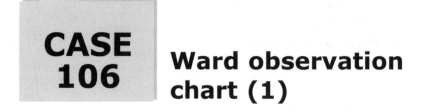

CASE 106

Ward observation chart (1)

Mr John Smith has a history of chronic liver failure due to alcohol abuse. He is admitted with abdominal distension, is feeling weak, and has been confused for two days. You are on ward duty from 11 to 14 January. During Mr Smith's admission, all observations have been recorded (see chart opposite).

1 Describe the pattern of abnormalities shown.

2 What is the most likely cause of these in this patient?

3 What symptoms will you ask about specifically?

4 What investigations will you request?

5 On 12 January Mr Smith feels very dizzy on sitting up. What action would you take?

6 He becomes very confused and drowsy. What complication would you suspect?

7 From 13 January what concerns you most about this patient's observations and why?

CASE
106

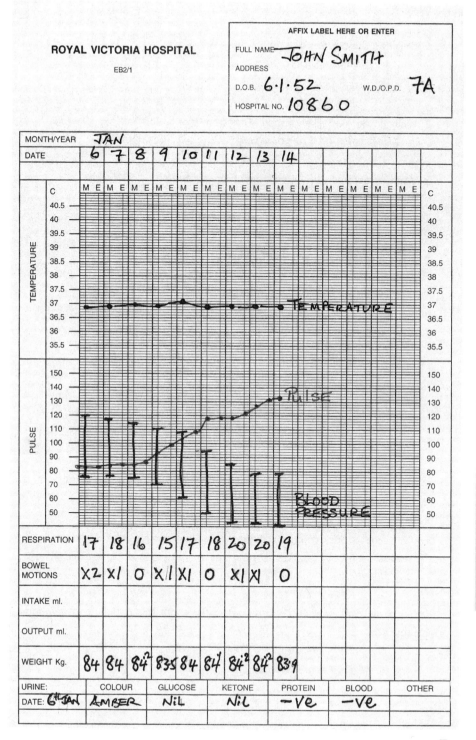

ROYAL VICTORIA HOSPITAL

EB2/1

AFFIX LABEL HERE OR ENTER

FULL NAME JOHN SMITH
ADDRESS
D.O.B. 6·1·52   W.D./O.P.D. 7A
HOSPITAL NO. 10860

MONTH/YEAR	JAN								
DATE	6	7	8	9	10	11	12	13	14

TEMPERATURE (C): 40.5, 40, 39.5, 39, 38.5, 38, 37.5, 37, 36.5, 36, 35.5

TEMPERATURE

PULSE: 150, 140, 130, 120, 110, 100, 90, 80, 70, 60, 50

PULSE

BLOOD PRESSURE

RESPIRATION	17	18	16	15	17	18	20	20	19
BOWEL MOTIONS	X2	X1	O	X/1	X1	O	X1	X1	O
INTAKE ml.									
OUTPUT ml.									
WEIGHT Kg.	84	84	84·2	83·5	84	84	84·2	84·2	83·9

URINE:	COLOUR	GLUCOSE	KETONE	PROTEIN	BLOOD	OTHER
DATE: 6th JAN	AMBER	NiL	NiL	−Ve	−Ve	

CASE 106

Answers

1 Describe the pattern of abnormalities shown.
- *Falling blood pressure*
- *Rising pulse rate.*

2 What is the most likely cause of these in this patient?
Gastrointestinal haemorrhage.

3 What symptoms will you ask about specifically?
- *Vomiting blood or coffee-grounds vomitus*
- *Melaena.*

4 What investigations will you request?
- *Full blood picture*
- *Blood group and crossmatch*
- *Urine and electrolytes*
- *Creatinine*
- *Coagulation screen*
- *Oesophagogastroduodenoscopy (OGD)*
- *Liver function tests.*

5 On 12 January Mr Smith feels very dizzy on sitting up. What action would you take?
- *Group and crossmatch blood*
- *Give intravenous fluids/blood.*

6 He becomes very confused and drowsy. What complication would you suspect?
Hepatic encephalopathy due to gastrointestinal haemorrhage.

7 From 13 January what concerns you most about this patient's observations and why?
- *Systolic pressure less than 80 mmHg*
- *Risk of acute renal failure.*

CASE
106

Data interpretation

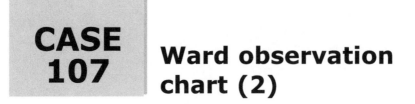

CASE 107 Ward observation chart (2)

Joseph Bloggs was admitted on 25 April following an episode of collapse. He has failed to regain consciousness, and all blood tests are normal. You are on ward duty from 26 to 29 April, during which time his level of consciousness is deteriorating. The observation chart for this patient is shown opposite.

1 What abnormalities are shown on the observation chart?

2 What does this pattern of change suggest to you as the likely cause of the unconsciousness?

3 List the most likely underlying possible causes in this patient.

4 What cranial nerve signs will you look for specifically?

5 What will you look for on examination of the fundus?

6 What investigation needs to be performed urgently?

CASE
107

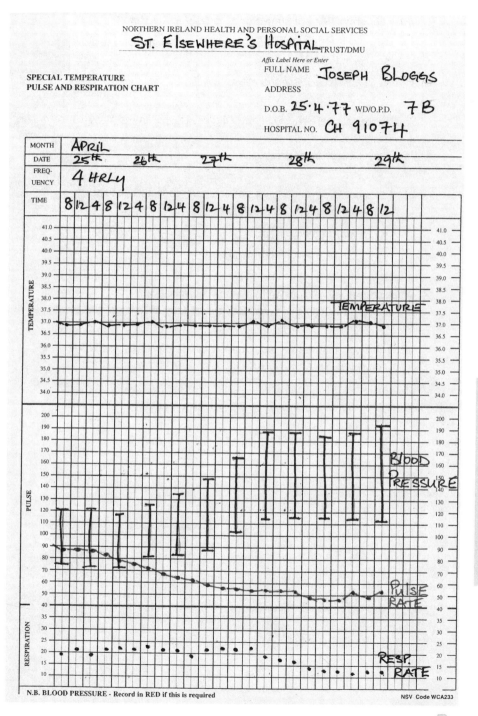

Answers

1 What abnormalities are shown on the observation chart?
- *Rising blood pressure*
- *Failing pulse*
- *Depressed respiratory rate.*

2 What does this pattern of change suggest to you as the likely cause of the unconsciousness?
   Rising intracranial pressure.

3 List the most likely underlying possible causes in this patient.
- *Haemorrhage (subarachnoid)*
- *Brain tumour*
- *Trauma with cerebral oedema.*

4 What cranial nerve signs will you look for specifically?
   Third nerve signs of constriction, and later dilation of the pupil.

5 What will you look for on examination of the fundus?
   Papilloedema.

6 What investigation needs to be performed urgently?
   CT scan of the brain.

Data interpretation

CASE
107

CASE 108

Ward observation chart (3)

Alison Jones was admitted with a history of fever and uncontrollable shivering which had been present intermittently for 48 hours. Despite oral penicillin therapy she remained very unwell. Examine the observation charts A and B opposite.

1 How would you describe the temperature pattern?

2 What are the most likely causes?

3 What complication developed on 19 March?

4 What condition has become apparent since 20 March?

5 If you were the house officer on duty, what fluid intake would you have permitted on 22 March?

6 What daily blood tests need to be requested?

7 What should the main treatment objective have been on the morning of 20 March?

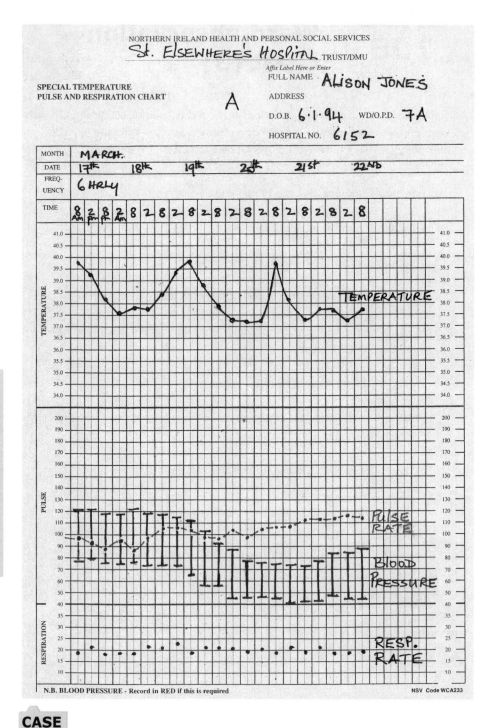

NORTHERN IRELAND HEALTH AND PERSONAL SOCIAL SERVICES

St. ElSEWHERE'S HOSPITAL TRUST/DMU

Affix Label Here or Enter

SPECIAL TEMPERATURE
PULSE AND RESPIRATION CHART   A

FULL NAME ALISON JONES

ADDRESS

D.O.B. 6·1·94   WD/O.P.D. 7A

HOSPITAL NO. 6152

MONTH	MARCH.					
DATE	17th	18th	19th	20th	21st	22nd
FREQ-UENCY	6 HRLY					

N.B. BLOOD PRESSURE - Record in RED if this is required   NSV Code WCA233

CASE
108

Data interpretation

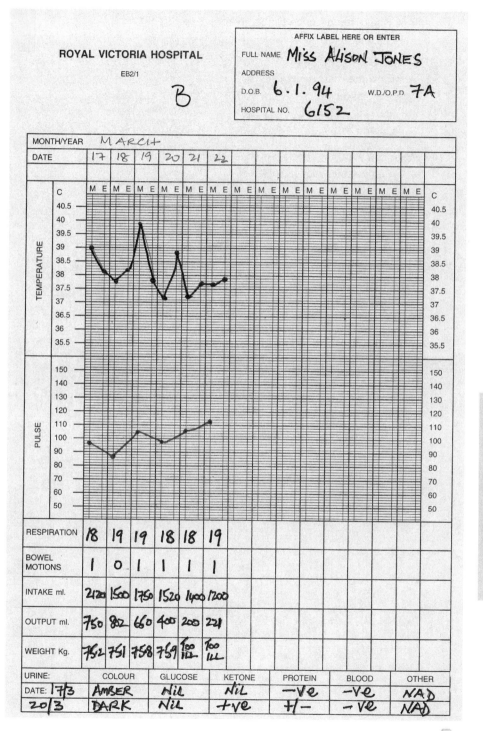

ROYAL VICTORIA HOSPITAL

EB2/1

B

AFFIX LABEL HERE OR ENTER

FULL NAME Miss Alison Jones

ADDRESS

D.O.B. 6.1.94   W.D./O.P.D. 7A

HOSPITAL NO. 6152

MONTH/YEAR	MARCH																							
DATE	17	18	19	20	21	22																		

RESPIRATION	18	19	19	18	18	19
BOWEL MOTIONS	1	0	1	1	1	1
INTAKE ml.	2120	1500	1750	1520	1400	1200
OUTPUT ml.	750	882	660	400	200	224
WEIGHT Kg.	752	751	758	759	700 / 112	700 / 112

URINE:	COLOUR	GLUCOSE	KETONE	PROTEIN	BLOOD	OTHER
DATE: 17/3	AMBER	Nil	Nil	−ve	−ve	NAD
20/3	DARK	Nil	+ve	+/−	−ve	NAD

Data interpretation

CASE 108

Answers

1 How would you describe the temperature pattern?
   Spiking fever.

2 What are the most likely causes?
   - *Abscess*
   - *Episodes of bacteraemia.*

3 What complication developed on 19 March?
   Septicaemia with hypotension.

4 What condition has become apparent since 20 March?
   Acute renal failure.

5 If you were the house officer on duty, what fluid intake would you have permitted on 22 March?
   700 ml.

6 What daily blood tests need to be requested?
   Electrolytes, urea and creatinine.

7 What should the main treatment objective have been on the morning of 20 March?
   To increase systolic blood pressure to > 80 mmHg.

CASE
108

CASE 109

Glucose tolerance testing

The graph below shows the results of glucose tolerance tests performed on three patients. After inspecting the graph, please answer the questions.

1 What is the diagnosis in patient A?

2 What are the two main criteria that you have used to reach this diagnosis?

3 What is the diagnosis in patient B?

4 Name two diseases which could be responsible for this result.

5 Glucose has been detected in the urine of patient C on more than one occasion. What is the likely cause of this?

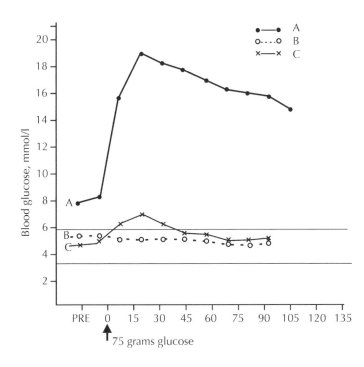

Data interpretation

Answers

1 What is the diagnosis in patient A?
    Diabetes mellitus.

2 What are the two main criteria that you have used to reach this diagnosis?
    • *Fasting blood sugar > 7 mmol/l*
    • *120-minute result > 11 mmol/l.*

3 What is the diagnosis in patient B?
    Malabsorption.

4 Name two diseases which could be responsible for this result.
    • *Coeliac disease*
    • *Crohn's disease.*

5 Glucose has been detected in the urine of patient C on more than one occasion. What is the likely cause of this?
    Low renal threshold for glucose.

Data interpretation

CASE
109

CASE 110

Pulmonary function tests (1)

A 70-year-old man complains of daily productive cough and exertional breathlessness. Look at his pulmonary function tests and answer the questions below.

	Measured	Predicted (%)
Forced expiratory volume in 1 second FEV_1	1.66 l	58
Forced vital capacity (FVC)	3.01 l	80
Peak expiratory flow rate (PEFR)	211 l/min	59
FEV_1/FVC	55%	80

1 What major abnormality of lung function does this represent?

2 What is the differential diagnosis?

3 What are the common aetiological factors?

4 What test might you perform to help to confirm the diagnosis?

5 What treatment would you recommend for the patient's cough and breathlessness?

Data interpretation

CASE
110

Answers

1 What major abnormality of lung function does this represent?
   Obstructive lung disease.

2 What is the differential diagnosis?
   - *Asthma*
   - *Chronic obstructive pulmonary disease (emphysema, chronic bronchitis).*

3 What are the common aetiological factors?
   - *Cigarette smoking*
   - *Air pollution*
   - *α_1-Antitrypsin deficiency.*

4 What test might you perform to help to confirm the diagnosis?
   - *Reversibility of pulmonary function tests with bronchodilator*
   - *Home peak expiratory flow rate monitoring*
   - *Trial of steroid therapy.*

5 What treatment would you recommend for the patient's cough and breathlessness?
   - *Inhaled bronchodilator*
   - *Oral bronchodilator.*

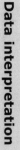

Data interpretation

CASE
110

CASE 111

Pulmonary function tests (2)

Pulmonary function tests were performed on two patients complaining of shortness of breath. The results (shown below) are expressed as percentages of those predicted for an age/sex-matched population of normal subjects.

	Patient A	Patient B
Forced vital capacity (FVC)	54%	71%
Forced expiratory volume in 1 second (FEV_1)	54%	44%
Peak expiratory flow rate (PEFR)	41%	58%
FEV_1/FVC	100%	63%

1 Which patient has obstructive lung disease?

2 Which patient is more likely to have normal total lung capacity?

3 Which patient could have cryptogenic fibrosing alveolitis?

4 What other lung function test would help to identify the patient with pulmonary fibrosis?

5 What other measurements would help to identify the patient with an obstructive lung disorder?

Data interpretation

CASE 111

Answers

1 Which patient has obstructive lung disease?
    Patient B.

2 Which patient is more likely to have normal total lung capacity?
    Patient B.

3 Which patient could have cryptogenic fibrosing alveolitis?
    Patient A.

4 What other lung function test would help to identify the patient with pulmonary fibrosis?
    Transfer factor.

5 What other measurements would help to identify the patient with an obstructive lung disorder?
    - *Reversibility studies ie pulmonary function tests before and after bronchodilators.*

Data interpretation

CASE
111

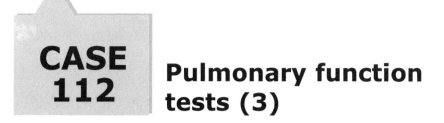

CASE 112

Pulmonary function tests (3)

Shown below are the results of pulmonary function tests that were obtained from a non-smoking patient with severe shortness of breath who has a dry cough.

	Percentage predicted
Forced vital capacity (FVC)	50%
Forced expiratory volume in 1 second (FEV_1)	49.5%
Peak expiratory flow rate (PEFR)	32%
FEV_1/FVC	98%
Carbon monoxide diffusing capacity	38%
(corrected for haemoglobin)	

1 What type of pulmonary disorder would cause these abnormal results?

2 Name two diseases which could cause this pattern of results.

3 What abnormality might be found on examination of the heart?

4 What might you expect to see on the chest X-ray?

5 On auscultation of the lung fields, what added sounds will be present?

Data interpretation

Answers

1 What type of pulmonary disorder would cause these abnormal results?
   A restrictive lung disease.

2 Name two diseases which could cause this pattern of results.
   - *Cryptogenic pulmonary fibrosis*
   - *Extrinsic allergic alveolitis*
   - *Sarcoidosis*
   - *Rheumatoid disease*
   - *Systemic lupus erythematosus*
   - *Ankylosing spondylitis.*

3 What abnormality might be found on examination of the heart?
   - *Left parasternal heave*
   - *Loud pulmonary second sound.*

4 What might you expect to see on the chest X-ray?
   Pulmonary fibrosis.

5 On auscultation of the lung fields, what added sounds will be present?
   Mid- to late-phase inspiratory crackles.

Data interpretation

CASE
112

Explanation/
communication

Explanation/communication

Marking overall score for communication stations

0	Unsatisfactory	Poor communication skills
		Rude or unsympathetic to the patient's questions
		Used medical jargon
		No organisation of subject material
1	Below average	Minor deficiencies in communication skills
		Did not clarify often
		Not fully organised or prepared when giving explanations
2	Satisfactory	Competent communicator
		Organised approach
		Well-structured, clear explanations
		Did not use medical jargon
		Occasionally gave patient the opportunity to ask questions and clarify points
3	Excellent	Highly competent communicator
		Well-organised, clear and easily understood explanations
		Very professional attitude and approach
		Gave patient plenty of opportunities to ask questions and clarify points

CASE 113

Testing for diabetes

Instructions for student

This patient has symptoms of polyuria and has been referred to the outpatient clinic for investigation of possible diabetes mellitus. Explain to the patient the various tests used to diagnose this condition, and describe the relative merits of each of them.

Instructions for examiner/simulated patient

You are a patient with symptoms of polyuria, and have been referred to the outpatient clinic for investigation of possible diabetes mellitus.

The student has been instructed to explain the various tests used to diagnose this condition, and to describe the relative merits of each of them.

Marking schedule

Adequate explanation of tests and their limitations.

Tests:

- urine analysis
- random sugar level
- fasting sugar level
- glucose tolerance test.

Limitations:

- urine analysis – why glycosuria does not necessarily indicate diabetes; low renal threshold for glucose
- random sugar level of > 11 mmol/l
- fasting blood sugar level of > 7 mmol/l
- glucose tolerance test – for borderline cases; how it is performed and how it is interpreted.

Overall score: 0   1   2   3   **(please circle one)**

CASE
113

Explanation/communication

CASE 114

Use of peak flow meter

Instructions for student

This patient has recently been diagnosed with asthma. Please instruct them in the use of a peak flow meter, and explain its role in the management of this condition.

Instructions for examiner/simulated patient

The student has been asked to instruct you in the use of a peak flow meter, and to explain its role in the management of asthma.

Marking schedule

Explanation of technique:

- patient standing
- indicator at zero
- breathe in/hold
- lips tight around the mouthpiece
- rapid expiration
- best of three recordings.

Potential uses of recordings:

- to show onset of attack and need to increase treatment
- to show effectiveness of treatment
- to detect precipitating or aggravating factors.

Overall score:　　　　**0**　　　**1**　　　**2**　　　**3**　　　　**(please circle one)**

CASE
114

CASE 115

Use of inhalers

Instructions for student

This patient has recently been diagnosed as having asthma and is to commence inhaled medication. Please instruct the patient in the correct use of salbutamol and becotide inhalers, and discuss the possible side effects of both drugs.

Explanation/communication

CASE
115

Instructions for examiner/simulated patient

The student has been asked to instruct you in the correct use of salbutamol and becotide inhalers, and to discuss the possible side effects of both drugs.

Marking schedule

Salbutamol – reliever.

Becotide – preventer.

Maximum frequency of use.

Side effects of salbutamol – tremor/palpitations.

Side effects of becotide – oral candidiasis, hoarseness.

Mouth rinse after use reduces risks.

Demonstration:

- to use while standing
- shake device before use
- co-ordination of inhalation and activation
- use of volumatic device (provided) if co-ordination is poor.

Overall score: 0   1   2   3   **(please circle one)**

CASE 115

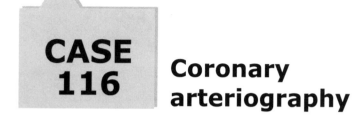

Coronary arteriography

Instructions for student

This patient has been diagnosed as having angina and requires coronary arteriography. Please inform them about:

- the nature of this investigation

- why it needs to be performed

- the risks of the procedure

- the medical treatment to be used if surgical therapy is not indicated.

Explanation/communication

CASE
116

Instructions for examiner/simulated patient

The student has been informed that you have angina and require coronary arteriography. They must explain:

- the nature of this investigation
- why it needs to be performed
- the risks of the procedure
- the medical treatment to be used if surgical therapy is not indicated.

Marking schedule

The nature of the investigation:

- explanation of technique – percutaneous, via inguinal approach, local anaesthetic
- explanation of what arteriography will demonstrate.

Why it needs to be performed:

To determine which intervention should be used – surgery/angioplasty with or without stent.

The risks of the procedure:

- haematoma
- false femoral aneurysm
- bleeding from site
- cardiac arrest, arrhythmia, myocardial infarction.

Medical treatments that can be used if surgical therapy is not indicated:

- aspirin
- nitrates
- ß-blockers
- statins
- calcium-channel blocking drugs.

Overall score: 0   1   2   3   **(please circle one)**

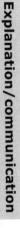
Explanation/communication

**CASE
116**

CASE 117

Oesophagogastroduo-denoscopy

Instructions for student

This patient has symptoms of dyspepsia. They need to have an oesophagogastroduo-denoscopy (OGD) performed.

Please inform them of the nature of this procedure, the information that may be obtained, and the complications or risks associated with the procedure.

Explanation/communication

CASE
117

Instructions for examiner/simulated patient

The student has been asked to explain how an OGD is performed, what information may be obtained, and the complications and risks associated with the procedure.

Marking schedule

Explanation of procedure:

- fasting
- sedation or topical anaesthetic administered to pharynx
- someone to accompany the patient (ie they must not drive home if sedated)
- what happens, with or without biopsy.

Information obtained:

- diseases of the oesophagus
- diseases of the stomach
- diseases of the duodenum.

Complications and risks:

- missed diagnosis
- perforation of the oesophagus
- haemorrhage.

Overall score: 0   1   2   3   **(please circle one)**

Explanation/communication

CASE
117

CASE 118

Starting anticoagulation

Instructions for student

This patient has a deep vein thrombosis in one leg and is to be started on anticoagulation therapy. Explain this method of treatment using warfarin; describe how drug therapy is initiated and monitored; and mention the important drug interactions that must be avoided.

Instructions for examiner/simulated patient

The student has been asked to explain anticoagulation treatment using warfarin, to describe how this drug therapy is initiated and monitored, and to mention the important drug interactions that must be avoided.

Please ask the student, 'Are there any golden rules about warfarin?' Then ask them about warning signs of an increased risk of bleeding.

Marking schedule

Method of treatment with warfarin – loading doses, then maintenance treatment.

How drug therapy will be monitored – regular visits to GP or anticoagulation clinic for blood tests to monitor international normalised ratio (INR).

Important drug interactions that must be avoided:

1 Increased risk of bleeding due to:
   - alcohol (especially binge drinking)
   - aspirin and aspirin-containing preparations
   - non-steroidal anti-inflammatory drugs (NSAIDs)
   - statins.

2 Reduced effectiveness of warfarin due to:
   - anti-epileptic drugs
   - oral contraceptive pill
   - steroids.

Golden rules:

Do not alter the amount of alcohol consumption, or start or stop any medication without first consulting a doctor. Always carry your anticoagulation card showing the dose of warfarin and INR results.

Warning signs of increased bleeding risk:

- bruising
- bleeding from gums
- nosebleeds
- blood in urine.

Overall score: 0   1   2   3   (please circle one)

Explanation/communication

CASE 118

CASE 119

Diet and fluid intake in chronic renal disease

Instructions for student

This patient has chronic renal failure as a result of chronic pyelonephritis. The urea concentration is 20.5 mmol/l (normal range 3.3–8.8 mmol/l) and the creatinine concentration is 350 μmol/l (normal range 40–110 μmol/l). Please give the patient advice about their diet and fluid balance, and then inform them of the symptoms they should look for which may develop as a complication of their condition.

Explanation/communication

Instructions for examiner/simulated patient

You are a patient with chronic renal failure (urea concentration 20.5 mmol/l and creatinine concentration of 350 μmol/l). The student must advise you about your diet and fluid intake. They must also inform you of symptoms which may develop as a complication of your condition.

Marking schedule

Advice about diet and fluid balance:

- low-protein, low-potassium diet (ie avoiding large quantities/portions of meat and fruit drinks and fruit, especially bananas)
- fluid intake volume should be approximately equivalent to the previous day's urinary volume output plus 500 ml. Never drink large volumes of fluid, as this may cause hypertension and/or pulmonary oedema.

Symptoms which would indicate the development of complications:

1 Symptoms of fluid overload:
   - shortness of breath
   - cough productive of frothy sputum
   - orthopnoea and paroxysmal nocturnal dyspnoea
   - oedema.

2 Symptoms of hypocalcaemia:
   - muscle weakness, tetany.

3 Symptoms of hyperkalaemia:
   - muscle paralysis.

4 Symptoms of uraemia:
   - nausea
   - vomiting
   - drowsiness
   - twitching.

Overall score: 0   1   2   3   **(please circle one)**

Explanation/communication

CASE
119

CASE 120

Hiatus hernia

Instructions for student

This patient has been diagnosed as having a hiatus hernia. Give them advice about the following:

- general measures they can take to relieve their symptoms

- the possible complications of this condition

- how the condition will be managed.

Instructions for examiner/simulated patient

You have a hiatus hernia. The student has been asked to give you advice about the general measures you can take to relieve your symptoms, the complications of this condition and how it will be managed.

Marking schedule

General measures:

Weight loss, small meals, not eating a meal before lying down, raising the head end of the bed by 1–2 inches.

Complications that can develop:

- stricture with symptoms of dysphagia
- Barrett's oesophagus.

Treatment used for this condition:

- weight-loss diet
- drugs to reduce or inhibit acid secretion in the stomach
- regular follow-up, with a repeat OGD every year if Barrett's oesophagus is present.

Overall score: 0   1   2   3   **(please circle one)**

Explanation/communication

CASE
120

Must-pass stations

Marking global performance score/rating for must-pass stations

0	Unsatisfactory	Major deficiencies in skills
		Unstructured approach
		Poor technique
1	Below average	Minor deficiencies in skills
		No systematic approach to skills
		Shows lack of experience or confidence in dealing with situation
2	Satisfactory	Competent in skills and professionalism
		Good approach, and shows some degree of organisation
		Considerate of patient safety
3	Excellent	Highly competent and professional
		Well organised and systematic
		Highly skilled in tasks

CASE 121

Basic life support

Instructions for student

You are called urgently back to a medical ward to see a patient who was admitted five days earlier having had a myocardial infarction. The nurse informs you that the patient has lost consciousness and is pale. When you enter this station the examiner will give further instructions.

Instructions for examiner

The candidate is required to demonstrate competence in basic life support using the BLS mannequin.

When the student enters the station, point to the mannequin and state, 'The patient has collapsed – I think they've had a cardiac arrest. Please do something quickly.'

Answers

Scoring	Not done/ inadequate	Properly performed
Check that the area is safe	☐	☐
Check patient's response to voice	☐	☐
Check patient's response to pain	☐	☐
Shout or send for help	☐	☐
Check airway (head tilt, chin lift, look in mouth)	☐	☐
Check for respirations for 10 sec (look, listen, feel)	☐	☐
Give two breaths by mouth-to-mouth ventilation	☐	☐
Check for pulse – 'none'	☐	☐
15 chest compressions	☐	☐
Repeat, ratio 2:15	☐	☐
Sequence – breaths then compressions? (please circle correct answer)	Yes	No
Does student need remedial training? (please circle correct answer)	Yes	No
Score for global performance: (please circle one)	0 1 2 3	

Comments for feedback/counselling:

CASE
121

CASE 122

Cardiac resuscitation

Instructions for student

Please enter this station. The examiner will instruct you on what action to take.

Instructions for examiner

The student must demonstrate how they would defibrillate a patient who has ventricular fibrillation. They do **not** need to perform basic life support. Say to the candidate, 'Thank goodness you've arrived! I've been giving mouth-to-mouth and cardiac massage – the arrest trolley is there but I don't know what to do. Please do something.'

CASE
122

Answers

Scoring	Not done/ inadequate	Properly performed
Establish ECG monitoring	☐	☐
Rhythm recognition – ventricular fibrillation	☐	☐
Correct position of paddles/pads	☐	☐
Check and instruct others to stand clear	☐	☐
Check rhythm before defibrillation	☐	☐
Shock 200 joules	☐	☐
Check rhythm between shocks	☐	☐
Shock 200 joules	☐	☐
Shock 360 joules	☐	☐
Recognise sinus rhythm	☐	☐
Check pulse/blood pressure	☐	☐

Correct sequence?   Yes   No
(please circle correct answer)

Was student competent?   Yes   No
(please circle correct answer)

Did student do anything dangerous?   Yes   No
(please circle correct answer)

Score for global performance: 0   1   2   3
(please circle one)

Comment for feedback/counselling:

Must-pass stations

CASE
122

CASE 123

Death certification

Instructions for student

At this station you must complete a death certificate for Mrs Jones, who you had been treating during her hospital admission, and who you certified dead on the ward.

The relevant history of her recent illness is provided. Please read the history carefully and complete the relevant sections of the death certificate. Sign it as if you were medically qualified to do so. For this purpose, put down your qualifications as MB, BCh, BAO and your address as St Elsewhere's Hospital, East Road, Homechester.

Mrs Alice Jones, 3 Main Road, Homechester, Unit Number 124316.

Mrs Jones, who had a 30-year history of non-insulin-dependent diabetes, was admitted eight days ago with a history of sudden onset of loss of power of the left arm and leg, together with loss of consciousness. CT scan confirmed the presence of a large area of infarction in the right cerebral hemisphere. Despite supportive therapy she made no significant signs of recovery. On the fourth day of her admission she developed fever, shortness of breath, and bilateral coarse crepitations were heard at the lung bases. Despite intravenous antibiotic therapy she failed to improve, became unresponsive, and died at 14.00 hours today. The family have been informed of Mrs Jones' death, and no post-mortem is necessary.

Must-pass stations

THIS CERTIFICATE MUST BE DELIVERED WITH THE DECEASED'S MEDICAL CARD WITHIN FIVE DAYS TO THE REGISTRAR FOR
THE DISTRICT IN WHICH THE PERSON (a) DIED OR   *FOR INSTRUCTIONS TO INFORMANTS*
(b) WAS ORDINARILY RESIDENT (WITHIN NORTHERN IRELAND) IMMEDIATELY BEFORE DEATH   *SEE OVERLEAF*

MEDICAL CERTIFICATE OF CAUSE OF DEATH

Births and Deaths Registration (Northern Ireland) Order 1976, Article 25(2)

To be signed by a Registered Medical Practitioner WHO HAS BEEN IN ATTENDANCE during the last
illness of the deceased person and given to some person required by Statute to give information of the death
to the Registrar. (SEE OVERLEAF)

FOR USE OF REGISTRAR
Entry No ....
District ....

Name of Deceased ....

Usual Residence ....

Place of Death ....

Date of Death .... day of .... 20 ......

Date on which last seen alive and treated by me for the undermentioned conditions .... day of .... 20 ......

Whether seen after death by me ....

Whether seen after death by another medical practitioner ....

	These particulars not to be entered in Death Register
CAUSE OF DEATH I	Approximate interval between onset and death (years, months, weeks, days, hours)
Disease or condition directly leading to death* (a).. due to (or as a consequence of)	....
Antecedent causes Morbid conditions, if any, giving rise to the above cause, stating the underlying condition last. (b)... due to (or as a consequence of) (c)...	
II	
Other significant conditions con-tributing to the death, but not related to the disease or condition causing it.	

*This does not mean the mode of dying eg heart failure, asthenia, etc. It means the disease, injury or complication which caused death.

I hereby certify that the above-named person has died as a result of the natural illness or disease for which he has been treated by me within twenty-eight
days prior to the date of death, and that the particulars and cause of death above written are true to the best of my knowledge and belief.

Signature ....

Residence ....

Qualifications as registered by General Medical Council ....

Date .... 20 ......

**The Health Service Number of the deceased should be entered here by the
certifying doctor.**

**CASE
123**

Answers

Name of deceased:

Date of death:

Date of certificate:

Place of death:

Cause of death: Ia   Bronchopneumonia – 4 days

               Ib   Intracerebral infarction – 8 days

               II   Non-insulin-dependent diabetes mellitus - 30 years

Form signed:

Name in block capitals:

Qualifications:

Residence:

Date completed:

Must-pass stations

CASE 123

CASE 124

Blood group and crossmatch request

Mr John Smith was admitted to Ward 6 as an acute medical emergency with a history of haematemesis and melaena. Mr Smith has been admitted under the consultant care of Dr FC Jones. The patients unit number is 85/123546 and his date of birth is 14/2/1928. On examination the patient is pale, sweating, pulse rate 115 beats per minute and blood pressure 90/60 and his haemoglobin is 7.2mmHg/dl. He had a previous episode of bleeding from a peptic ulcer on 1 April 1997 when he was given two units of packed red cells without any adverse reaction. Please complete the questions below.

Circle the correct answers and complete the laboratory request form.

1 What intravenous fluid will you request?

5% dextrose   Packed red cells

Fresh plasma

2 Which laboratory will you send the request form to?

Biochemistry   Coagulation laboratory

Bacteriology   Blood bank

3 What type of blood sample will you send?

Clotted blood   Heparin and blood

EDTA sample

4 You are very busy with other patients on the ward. Who can take the sample of blood for you?

The student nurse   Sister/charge nurse

A medical student   No one

CASE 124

5 How many units will you request?

2   6   12

6 Please complete the request form shown below.

BLOOD TRANSFUSION		
ATTACH LABEL OR USE BALL POINT PEN		WARD / CONSULTANT REQUIRED EVEN WITH LABEL

HOSPITAL No.

SURNAME

FORENAMES

DATE OF SPECIMEN

TIME OF SPECIMEN

CAT 3   **PRIVATE**

Belfast Link Labs

FOR LABORATORY USE ONLY

SEX   DATE OF BIRTH
M ☐ F ☐   ☐☐ / ☐☐ / ☐☐

CONSULTANT   SOURCE / WARD

Diagnosis / Reason for Transfusion
(state type of operation-ref Maximum Blood Order schedule)

BLOOD BANK

Group / Antibody Screen (Plasma Held Seven Days)   ☐

Direct Antiglobulin Test (Coombs Test)   ☐

Kleihauer Test   ☐

Crossmatch red cells units   No. of Units ☐

Special requirements _____

Other Requests _____

Required for: Date _____ Time _____ Deliver To _____

Product requested by: M.O's Signature _____

For Emergency requests, FFP, Cryo or Platelets please telephone blood bank
See Laboratory handbook for details of Maximum Blood Order Schedule.

Transfusion History

Blood group (if known): _____

Atypical antibodies (if known) _____

Previous transfusions   YES   NO

If YES date of last transfusion _____

Previous reactions   YES   NO

Previous pregnancies   YES   NO

Anti D given recently (<12 weeks)   YES   NO

I confirm that these patient identification details correspond to
the details of the patient and the specimen tube

Sample taken by: _____ Date _____

CASE
124

Answers

1 What intravenous fluid will you request?
   Packed red cells.

2 Which laboratory will you send the request form to?
   The blood bank.

3 What type of blood sample will you send?
   EDTA sample.

4 You are very busy with other patients on the ward. Who can take the
   sample of blood for you?
   No one.

5 How many units will you request?
   6

6 Request form must be completed and correct.

Hospital number	85/123546
Surname	Smith
Forename	John
Gender	Male
Date of birth	14/02/28
Consultant	Dr FC Jones
Ward	6
Date of specimen	–/–/–
Time	24-hour clock
Diagnosis	Haematemesis/melaena
Request	6 units of packed red cells
Date	–/–/–
Time	Soon after request
Deliver to	Ward 6
Signature	Must be signed
Blood group	Not known
Previous transfusion	Yes
Date	1/4/97
Sample taken by	Student's name
Date	As above

Must-pass stations

CASE
124

CASE 125

Management of diabetic coma

Part A

Miss Jane Stevens is a 24-year-old university student who has a ten-year history of insulin-dependent diabetes mellitus. She is admitted to the Accident and Emergency Department having been found collapsed in her kitchen. Her flatmate states that Miss Stevens was well earlier that morning but must have collapsed while preparing breakfast.

1 What is the most likely cause of the patient's loss of consciousness?

2 Given that the treatments listed below are appropriate for the clinical situation, please rank them (from 1–7) to show the sequence of actions that you would take.
   - Give oral glucose solution
   - Flush cannula with 0.9% saline
   - Give 50 ml of 50% dextrose intravenously
   - Erect a 10% dextrose infusion
   - Send blood sample to laboratory for glucose assay
   - Check blood glucose level with glucometer
   - Check dose of insulin by asking the patient.

CASE
125

Part A Answers

1 What is the most likely cause of the patient's loss of consciousness?
      Hypoglycaemia.

2 Given that the treatments listed below are appropriate for the clinical situation, please rank them (from 1–7) to show the sequence of actions that you would take.

   • *Give oral glucose solution*   *(6)*
   • *Flush cannula with 0.9% saline*   *(3)*
   • *Give 50 ml of 50% dextrose intravenously*   *(2)*
   • *Erect a 10% dextrose infusion*   *(5)*
   • *Send blood sample to laboratory for glucose assay* *(4)*
   • *Check blood glucose level with glucometer*   *(1)*
   • *Check dose of insulin by asking the patient*   *(7)*

**CASE
125**

Part B

Two weeks later Miss Stevens is admitted deeply unconscious. Her flatmate informs you that she had been unwell for two days with fever, cough and slight shortness of breath. Miss Stevens had not been eating her meals regularly, and her flatmate is unsure whether or not she was taking her insulin.

1 What is the most likely cause of the patient's loss of consciousness?

2 What are the four main principles of management of this condition?

3 Given that the treatments listed below are appropriate for the clinical condition, please rank them (from 1–5) to show the sequence of actions that you would take within the first 30 minutes.
   - Send blood samples to the laboratory for blood glucose, full blood picture and biochemistry
   - Start intravenous antibiotic therapy
   - Erect 1 litre of 0.9% saline and infuse over 20 minutes
   - Estimate blood sugar level with glucometer
   - Give 10 units of soluble insulin intravenously

4 What investigations should be repeated every hour on this patient until her condition is thought to be safe?

5 What volume of fluid should be infused in the first 24 hours?
   (circle the correct answer)

   2 litres   3 litres   6 litres   18 litres

6 If the blood sugar level is elevated during this time, how frequently and by what route is insulin administered? (tick the correct answer)

   ☐   Hourly by subcutaneous injection

   ☐   Every two hours by intravenous injection

   ☐   Every 15 minutes by intramuscular injection

   ☐   Every hour by intramuscular injection

   ☐   Every 15 minutes by intravenous injection

Must-pass stations

CASE
125

Part B Answers

1 What is the most likely cause of the patient's loss of consciousness?
    Hyperglycaemia/ketoacidosis.

2 What are the four main principles of management of this condition?
    - *Fluid replacement*
    - *Insulin administration*
    - *Electrolyte and acid–base balance*
    - *Treatment of underlying cause.*

3 Given that the treatments listed below are appropriate for the clinical condition, please rank them (from 1–5) to show the sequence of actions that you would take within the first 30 minutes.
    - *Send blood samples to the laboratory for blood glucose, full blood picture and biochemistry*   *(2)*
    - *Start intravenous antibiotic therapy*   *(5)*
    - *Erect 1 litre of 0.9% saline and infuse over 20 minutes*   *(3)*
    - *Estimate blood sugar level with glucometer*   *(1)*
    - *Give 10 units of soluble insulin intravenously*   *(4)*

4 What investigations should be repeated every hour on this patient until her condition is thought to be safe?
    - *Blood sugar*
    - *Serum potassium*
    - *pH of blood.*

5 What volume of fluid should be infused in the first 24 hours?
    6 litres.

6 If the blood sugar level is elevated during this time, how frequently and by what route is insulin administered?
    Every hour by intramuscular injection.

CASE 125

CASE 126

Anaphylactic shock

You are called to attend the medical ward urgently to see a 20-year-old male patient who has developed swelling of the lips and tongue 15 minutes after receiving 500 mg of penicillin V medication, which was given intravenously.

1 What name is given to the soft tissue swelling of the lips and tongue?

2 What questions would you ask the patient?

3 What clinical signs would you specifically look for on examination?

4 The patient is not distressed and their vital signs are normal. What drug treatment would you consider giving?

5 The patient's condition suddenly deteriorates with more marked swelling of the face and development of a generalised erythematous rash and stridor. The blood pressure falls to 60/20 mmHg and the patient becomes cyanosed. What name is given to this clinical state?

6 What type of hypersensitivity reaction causes this condition?

7 What treatment would you administer?

8 The patient improves within 4–5 minutes, but his blood pressure remains low at 70/40 mmHg. What action would you take?

9 The condition of the patient improves and his blood pressure is now 110/60 mmHg. What observations would you request the nursing staff to record over the next 12 hours?

10 What amendments would you make to the drug chart?

CASE
126

Answers

1 What name is given to the soft tissue swelling of the lips and tongue?
     Angio-oedema.

2 What questions would you ask the patient?
   - *Are you allergic to penicillin?*
   - *Do you feel short of breath?*
   - *Have you any difficulty with swallowing?*
   - *Do you feel faint or dizzy?*
   - *Do you have chest pain or palpitations?*

3 What clinical signs would you specifically look for on examination?
   - *Tachycardia*
   - *Hypotension*
   - *Respiratory wheeze or stridor*
   - *Cyanosis.*

4 The patient is not distressed and their vital signs are normal. What drug
   treatment would you consider giving?
   - *Oral antihistamine (eg Piriton® 4 mg eight-hourly)*
   - *Oral corticosteroid.*

5 The patient's condition suddenly deteriorates with more marked swelling of
   the face and development of a generalised erythematous rash and stridor.
   The blood pressure falls to 60/20 mmHg and the patient becomes cyanosed.
   What name is given to this clinical state?
     Anaphylactic shock.

6 What type of hypersensitivity reaction causes this condition?
     Type I – IgE-mediated reaction.

7 What treatment would you administer?
   - *100% oxygen by inhalation*
   - *0.5 ml of 1 in 1000 adrenaline (epinephrine) intramuscularly*
   - *10 mg of Piriton® (chlorpheniramine) intravenously*
   - *250 mg of hydrocortisone intravenously.*

**CASE
126**

8 The patient improves within 4–5 minutes, but his blood pressure remains low at 70/40 mmHg. What action would you take?
- *Give 0.5 ml of 1 in 1000 adrenaline intramuscularly*
- *Erect intravenous infusion.*

9 The condition of the patient improves and his blood pressure is now 110/60 mmHg. What observations would you request the nursing staff to record over the next 12 hours?
- *Pulse rate*
- *Blood pressure*
- *Respiratory rate.*

10 What amendments would you make to the drug chart?
- *Stop penicillin V and change to a non-penicillin antibiotic*
- *Chlorpheniramine, 4–8 mg eight-hourly, intravenously or orally*
- *Hydrocortisone, 100–300 mg six-hourly, intravenously*
- *Record 'allergic to pencillin'.*

Must-pass stations

CASE
126

Therapeutics and pharmacology

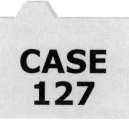

CASE 127

The hypertensive patient

Drug chart

Drug	Dose	Route	Frequency
1 Salbutamol	2.5 mg	Nebuliser	Three times daily
2 Ipratropium bromide	250 micrograms	Nebuliser	Three times daily
3 Amiloride	5 mg	Oral	Once daily
4 Slow-K (potassium chloride)	2 tabs	Oral	Twice daily
5 Metoprolol	100 mg	Oral	Twice daily
6 Captopril	50 mg	Oral	Once daily

A patient was admitted to hospital with a past history of hypertension which was poorly controlled. Over a period of six months he had been started on drugs 3, 5 and then 6 (see drug chart) to achieve control of his hypertension. After a few weeks he developed a cough, and the family doctor prescribed drugs 1 and 2. On a routine blood test he was found to have a slightly low potassium level, and drug 4 was commenced.

On examination the patient has a tremor, some shortness of breath with wheeze, and a pulse rate of 40 beats per minute. The results of biochemical tests show raised urea and creatinine levels and a serum potassium concentration of 5.8 mmol/l.

1 Which of the drugs listed can cause a tremor?
2 Which of the drugs can cause impaired renal function?
3 Which drug can cause a troublesome dry cough?
4 Which drugs could be contributing to the raised serum potassium level?
5 Which drug causes bradycardia?
6 Which drug can cause tachycardia?
7 Which drug should not be prescribed for a patient with obstructive lung disease?
8 Which of the drugs can cause hypokalaemia?

Answers

1 Which of the drugs listed can cause a tremor?

(1) Salbutamol.

2 Which of the drugs can cause impaired renal function?

(3) Amiloride

(6) Captopril.

3 Which drug can cause a troublesome dry cough?

(6) Captopril.

4 Which drugs could be contributing to the raised serum potassium level?

(3) Amiloride

(4) Slow-K

(6) Captopril.

5 Which drug causes bradycardia?

(5) Metoprolol.

6 Which drug can cause tachycardia?

(1) Salbutamol.

7 Which drug should not be prescribed for a patient with obstructive lung disease?

(5) Metoprolol.

8 Which of the drugs can cause hypokalaemia?

(1) Salbutamol.

CASE
127

CASE 128

The hypertensive patient with asthma

A patient is admitted with fever, shortness of breath and a productive cough. There is a past history of penicillin allergy, high blood pressure and asthma. His drug therapy on admission is as follows:

- salbutamol inhaler, two puffs three times daily
- ipratropium bromide inhaler, two puffs three times daily
- bendroflumethiazide (bendrofluazide), 5 mg orally once daily
- propranolol, 40 mg orally three times daily
- theophylline, 275 mg orally three times daily
- the locum GP recommended starting ampicillin, 500 mg three times daily, but the patient has been unable to get to the pharmacy with his prescription.

1 Of the six drugs prescribed for this patient, which will you **not** prescribe while he is in hospital?

2 Name two of the drugs which can cause hypokalaemia.

3 Which drug can cause hyperglycaemia?

4 Which drug should not be prescribed for a patient with asthma?

5 Which of the drugs can cause convulsions if the serum level is too high?

6 What blood test could be done to confirm the diagnosis of penicillin allergy?

CASE
128

Answers

1 Of the six drugs prescribed for this patient, which will you not prescribe
    while he is in hospital?
    - *Propranolol*
    - *Ampicillin.*

2 Name two of the drugs which can cause hypokalaemia.
    - *Salbutamol*
    - *Bendroflumethiazide.*

3 Which drug can cause hyperglycaemia?
    Bendroflumethiazide.

4 Which drug should not be prescribed for a patient with asthma?
    Propranolol.

5 Which of the drugs can cause convulsions if the serum level is too high?
    Theophylline.

6 What blood test could be done to confirm the diagnosis of penicillin allergy?
    RAST to penicillin.

CASE
128

CASE 129

The diabetic patient with urinary infection

A 62-year-old type 2 diabetic patient is admitted with symptoms of a urinary tract infection and nausea. On admission her drug therapy is as follows:

- co-trimoxazole (Septrin®), 960 mg twice daily
- cyclopenthiazide (Navidrex®), 500 micrograms once daily
- metformin, 500 mg three times daily
- metoclopramide (Maxolon®), 20 mg three times daily.

1 Which one of these drugs could worsen control of blood glucose levels?

2 What blood test could be performed to assess control of blood sugar levels?

3 Which of these drugs could cause a fall in the white cell count (neutropenia)?

4 During the three days of her admission the patient develops abnormal movements of her arms and face. Which drug is most likely to be responsible for this movement disorder?

5 What name is given to this abnormality?

6 Which two drugs should not be used in patients with liver or renal impairment?

7 Which drug predisposes to lactic acidosis?

8 Which drug causes hypokalaemia?

CASE
129

Answers

1 Which one of these drugs could worsen control of blood glucose levels?
   Cyclopenthiazide.

2 What blood test could be performed to assess control of blood sugar levels?
   Hb A_{1C}.

3 Which of these drugs could cause a fall in the white cell count (neutropenia)?
   Co-trimoxazole.

4 During the three days of her admission the patient develops abnormal movements of her arms and face. Which drug is most likely to be responsible for this movement disorder?
   Metoclopramide.

5 What name is given to this abnormality?
   Tardive dyskinesia.

6 Which two drugs should not be used in patients with liver or renal impairment?
   • *Metformin*
   • *Metoclopramide.*

7 Which drug predisposes to lactic acidosis?
   Metformin.

8 Which drug causes hypokalaemia?
   Cyclopenthiazide.

CASE
129

CASE 130

Chronic obstructive lung disease

A patient with a long history of chronic bronchitis is admitted with an acute exacerbation. He has recently been started on a course of oral steroids. His full list of medication is as follows:

- prednisolone, 60 mg once daily
- salbutamol inhaler, two puffs four times daily
- ephedrine hydrochloride, 30 mg three times daily
- theophylline, 300 mg twice daily.

On examination, the patient has widespread expiratory wheezes. His pulse rate is 120 beats per minute, he has a marked tremor and his blood pressure is 170/105 mmHg.

1 What concentration of oxygen would you give by inhalation?

2 Why would you not give 100% oxygen?

3 Before giving the patient intravenous aminophylline to relieve his shortness of breath, what would you do?

4 At what rate would you give the aminophylline injection (in ml/minute)?

5 Which drugs are contributing to his tachycardia?

6 Which drugs are contributing to his high blood pressure?

7 List four side effects of prednisolone.

CASE 130

Answers

1 What concentration of oxygen would you give by inhalation?
    28%.

2 Why would you not give 100% oxygen?
    In patients with chronic obstructive pulmonary disease, the respiratory centre relies on the low oxygen level for respiratory stimulation.

3 Before giving the patient intravenous aminophylline to relieve his shortness of breath, what would you do?
    Check the serum theophylline level.

4 At what rate would you give the aminophylline injection (in ml/minute)?
    1 ml/minute.

5 Which drugs are contributing to his tachycardia?
    • *Salbutamol*
    • *Ephedrine hydrochloride.*

6 Which drugs are contributing to his high blood pressure?
    • *Ephedrine hydrochloride*
    • *Prednisolone.*

7 List four side effects of prednisolone.
    • *Hypertension*
    • *Psychosis*
    • *Adrenal failure*
    • *Osteoporosis*
    • *Myopathy*
    • *Weight gain*
    • *Infection*
    • *Peptic ulceration*
    • *Pulmonary oedema*
    • *Avascular necrosis*
    • *Cushing's syndrome*
    • *Hyperglycaemia.*

CASE
130

CASE 131

The patient after myocardial infarction

A patient with a past history of hypertension had an acute myocardial infarction five days ago. He is ready for discharge and has been prescribed five drugs. For each drug, give the main indication for use and two side effects which could develop.

1   Aspirin, 300 mg once daily.

2   Atenolol, 50 mg once daily.

3   Captopril, 50 mg twice daily.

4   Pravastatin, 20 mg at night.

5   Bendroflumethiazide (bendrofluazide), 5 mg once daily.

CASE
131

Answers

1   Aspirin, 300 mg once daily.

> *Reason for use:* to reduce risk of thrombosis
>
> *Side effects:* • *gastric erosions*
>
> • *bronchospasm*
>
> • *bleeding.*

2   Atenolol, 50 mg once daily.

> *Reason for use:* anti-anginal/hypertension
>
> *Side effects:* • *lethargy*
>
> • *peripheral vascular ischaemia*
>
> • *impotence.*

3   Captopril, 50 mg twice daily.

> *Reason for use:* hypertension/heart failure
>
> *Side effects:* • *first dose – postural hypotension*
>
> • *cough.*

4   Pravastatin, 20 mg at night.

> *Reason for use:* to reduce lipid levels
>
> *Side effects:* • *gastrointestinal upset*
>
> • *chest pain*
>
> • *fatigue*
>
> • *abnormal liver function tests*
>
> • *muscle pain.*

5   Bendroflumethiazide, 5 mg once daily.

> *Reason for use:* hypertension/to prevent left ventricular failure (LVF)
>
> *Side effects:* • *increased blood sugar level*
>
> • *hypokalaemia.*

CASE
131

CASE 132

Congestive heart failure and atrial fibrillation

A patient with congestive heart failure and fast atrial fibrillation (pulse rate 120 beats per minute) has been started on three drugs. For each drug, give the indication for use, state the mechanism of action and list two side effects.

1 Digoxin, 250 micrograms once daily.

2 Furosemide (frusemide), 40 mg once daily.

3 Warfarin, 3 mg once daily.

CASE
132

Answers

For each drug, give the indication for use, state the mechanism of action and list two side effects.

1 Digoxin, 250 micrograms once daily.

> *Reason for use: to control ventricular rate*

> *Mechanism of action: slows conduction at atrioventricular node/positive inotrope*

> *Side effects:* • *nausea*
> • *heart block*
> • *bradycardia.*

2. Furosemide, 40 mg once daily.

> *Reason for use: congestive cardiac failure*

> *Mechanism of action: prevents sodium and water resorption in loop of Henle*

> *Side effects:* • *hypokalaemia*
> • *hyponatraemia*
> • *acute urinary retention*
> • *increased uric acid levels.*

3. Warfarin, 3 mg once daily.

> *Reason for use: to prevent thrombus formation in the left atrium*

> *Mechanism of action: reduces levels of vitamin K-dependent clotting factors*

> *Side effects:* • *haemorrhage*
> • *skin rash*
> • *liver dysfunction*
> • *alopecia.*

**CASE
132**

CASE 133

A diabetic patient with heart failure and COPD

For each of the drugs listed below, give the mode of action and name one common medical condition for which the drug is prescribed.

1 Gliclazide (class: sulphonylurea).

2 Isosorbide mononitrate (class: nitrate).

3 Furosemide (frusemide) (class: loop diuretic).

4 Lisinopril (class: ACE inhibitor).

5 Salbutamol inhaler (class: β_2-agonist).

CASE
133

Answers

1 Gliclazide (class: sulphonylurea).

> *Mode of action: increases insulin production from the pancreas*
>
> *Indication: type 2 diabetes.*

2 Isosorbide mononitrate (class: nitrate).

> *Mode of action: vasodilator*
>
> *Indication: angina.*

3 Furosemide (class: loop diuretic).

> *Mode of action: decreases sodium and water resorption*
>
> *Indication: cardiac failure/oedema.*

4 Lisinopril (class: ACE inhibitor).

> *Mode of action: vasodilator (inhibits conversion of angiotensin I to angiotensin II)*
>
> *Indications: heart failure/hypertension.*

5 Salbutamol inhaler (class: β_2-agonist).

> *Mode of action: bronchodilation by stimulation of β_2-receptors*
>
> *Indications: asthma/chronic obstructive pulmonary disease.*

CASE 133

CASE 134

Drug chart with errors (1)

This drug chart contains a number of errors. Please make a note of five serious errors.

Start date 1/1/03

The ROYAL
HOSPITALS

Drug Prescription and Administration Record (DPAR1)

03/45291.
MR FREDERICK FLINTSTONE

~~Patient details~~
~~Affix label~~

3 JELLYSTONE PARK
ROCKVILLE.

Drug allergies:

PENICILLIN ALLERGY

Weight 95 Kg   Date 1.1.03   Signature [signature]
Weight   Date   Signature

For the safety of the patient, please read the following instructions:
- Use generic names;
- Do not alter existing instructions;
- Discontinue a drug by drawing a line through it and signing.
- All drugs given must be initialled in the appropriate box.
- Write in CAPITALS and BLACK ink;
- Changes must be ordered by a new prescription;

REGULAR PRESCRIPTIONS

Date, month and year →	Times ↓	1/1	2/1	3/1	4/1	5/1	6/1			
Drug SPIRONOLACTONE Frequency bd	0800									
Dose 200 Route O Start date 1/1/03 Stop date										
Signature Stop signature	1600									
Additional information	2000									
Drug SLOW K Frequency bd	0800									
Dose TT Route O Start date 1/1/03 Stop date										
Signature Stop signature										
Additional information	1600									
Drug AMPICILLIN Frequency QID	0800									
Dose 500mg Route O Start date 1/1/03 Stop date	1200									
Signature Stop signature	1600									
Additional information FOR 7 DAYS	2800									
Drug CAPOTEN Frequency bd	0800									
Dose 25m Route O Start date Stop date										
Signature Stop signature										
Additional information	2000									
Drug Frequency	8Am									
Dose 80mg Route O Start date 1/1/08 Stop date										
Signature Stop signature										
Additional information	10pm									

WMX 2139 011648

CASE 134

Answers

- *Three drugs that increase potassium levels.*
- *Slow-K has no signature.*
- *Patient is allergic to penicillin but is on ampicillin x 2.*
- *Non-generic prescription.*
- *Inderal – drug name is illegible.*
- *No start date for Capoten®.*
- *Excessive dose of spironolactone.*
- *Spironolactone prescribed twice a day but given three times daily.*

Therapeutics and pharmacology

CASE
134

CASE 135

Drug chart with errors (2)

This drug chart contains a number of errors. Please make a note of five errors or problems with the drugs prescribed.

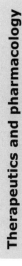

The **ROYAL**
HOSPITALS

Start date

Drug Prescription and Administration Record (DPAR1)

03/275291

MR BERNARD RUBBLE
~~Patient details~~
~~Affix label~~
1 JELLYSTONE PARK
ROCKVILLE

Drug allergies:

NONE

Weight 59 Kg   Date 1/1/03   Signature

For the safety of the patient, please read the following instructions:
- Use generic names;
- Do not alter existing instructions;
- Discontinue a drug by drawing a line through it and signing.
- All drugs given must be initialled in the appropriate box.
- Write in CAPITALS and BLACK ink;
- Changes must be ordered by a new prescription;

REGULAR PRESCRIPTIONS

Date, month and year →	Times ↓	1/1	2/1	3/1	4/1	5/1	6/1						
Drug SALBUTAMOL Frequency t.i.d.	0800	MV	M.	MN									
Dose 2.5mg Route NEB Start date 1/1 Stop date	1600	MV	MV										
Signature Stop signature	2000	MV	Mr										
Additional information													
Drug ATROVENT Frequency t.d.	0800	m	m	m									
Dose 250 mcg Route NEB Start date 1/1 Stop date	1600	m	m										
Signature Stop signature	2000	L	L										
Additional information													
Drug PROPRANOLOL Frequency t.d.	0800	m	m	m									
Dose 40mg Route O Start date Stop date													
Signature Stop signature	2000	m	L										
Additional information													
Drug _____ Frequency t.d.	8AM	m	m	N									
Dose 275mg Route O Start date 1/1/03 Stop date													
Signature Stop signature	10pm	✗											
Additional information													
Drug AMILORIDE Frequency OD	0800	✗	✗	✗									
Dose 5mg Route O Start date 1/1/03 Stop date													
Signature Stop signature													
Additional information													

WMX 2139 011648

CASE 135

Answers

- *Illegible writing (theophylline).*
- *Non-generic prescription (Atrovent®).*
- *Dosage regime given incorrectly (Atrovent®).*
- *No signature (amiloride).*
- *β-Blocker (propranolol) used in a patient with obstructive airways disease.*

Therapeutics and pharmacology

CASE
135

CASE 136

Myocardial infarction

Three drugs commonly used to treat patients following a myocardial infarction are listed below. For each drug please list the reason for use, the usual dose for an 80 kg adult patient, the route of administration used to treat acute myocardial infarction, and a major side effect.

1 Diamorphine.

2 Cyclizine.

3 Furosemide (frusemide).

Answers

1 Diamorphine.

> *Reason for use: analgesia*
>
> *Dose: 2.5–5 mg*
>
> *Route of administration: intravenous*
>
> *Side effects:* • *nausea and vomiting*
>
> • *respiratory depression.*

2 Cyclizine.

> *Reason for use: anti-emetic*
>
> *Dose: 50 mg*
>
> *Route of administration: intravenous or oral*
>
> *Side effect: drowsiness.*

3 Furosemide (frusemide).

> *Reason for use: diuretic*
>
> *Dose: 40 mg*
>
> *Route of administration: intravenous*
>
> *Side effect: potassium depletion*
>
> • *urinary retention.*

CASE
136

CASE 137

Cardiovascular disease

For each of the following drugs, please list an indication for use, adult dose, side effect, contraindication and drug interaction.

1 Digoxin.

2 Atenolol.

3 Verapamil.

Answers

1 Digoxin.

> *Indication: atrial fibrillation*
>
> *Dose: 62.5–500 micrograms*
>
> *Side effects:* • *nausea*
>
>   • *yellow vision*
>
> *Contraindications: first- or second-degree heart block*
>
> *Drug interactions: ß-blockers/amiodarone.*

2 Atenolol.

> *Indications: angina/ hypertension*
>
> *Dose: 25–100 mg daily*
>
> *Side effect: bradycardia*
>
> *Contraindications: peripheral vascular disease, chronic obstructive pulmonary disease*
>
> *Drug interactions: verapamil, calcium-channel blockers.*

3 Verapamil.

> *Indication: supraventricular tachycardia*
>
> *Dose: 40–120 mg three times a day*
>
> *Side effect: heart failure*
>
> *Contraindications: hypotension, bradycardia, heart block*
>
> *Drug interaction: ß-blockers.*

Therapeutics and pharmacology

CASE 137

CASE 138

Reflux oesophagitis

Reflux oesophagitis is a common medical condition. List three drugs which can be used to treat the symptoms, state the usual dose, and give one important side effect or complication which can occur with treatment.

Answers

Check individual student answers with *British National Formulary* drugs for
dyspepsia:

- *antacids*
- *proton-pump inhibitors*
- *H₂-blockers.*

For example:

Name of drug: omeprazole
Dose: 10–40 mg daily
Side effect/complication: dry mouth.

**CASE
138**

CASE 139

Analgesic prescribing

Pain is an extremely common symptom. List three analgesics which you would prescribe, noting the dose, route of administration, frequency of use and one important side effect.

1 Analgesic for mild to moderate pain.

2 Analgesic for moderately severe pain.

3 Analgesic for severe pain.

Answers

Check individual student answers with *British National Formulary* 'pain' or 'analgesic' sections.

Examples:

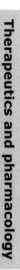

1 Analgesic for mild to moderate pain.

Drug name	*Paracetamol*
Dose	*0.5–1.0 g*
Route of administration	*Oral*
Frequency of use	*Four to six hourly*
Side effect	*Liver damage if given in excess*

2 Analgesic for moderately severe pain.

Drug name	*Dihydrocodeine*
Dose	*30 mg*
Route of administration	*Oral*
Frequency of use	*Every four to six hours*
Side effects	*Hypotension, tachycardia*

3 Analgesic for severe pain.

Drug name	*Diamorphine hydrochloride*
Dose	*5–10 mg*
Route of administration	*Subcutaneous, intramuscular or intravenous*
Frequency of use	*Every four hours if needed*
Side effect	*Nausea, vomiting/respiratory depression*

CASE
139

CASE 140

Deep vein thrombosis

Describe the principles of treatment of deep vein thrombosis (DVT) in a patient with no previous history of DVT and no contraindications or complicating factors.

1 What form of drug therapy is used for the initial management?
   - Name of the drug
   - Approximate dose for a 60 kg patient
   - Route of administration
   - Frequency of treatment per day.

2 What drug therapy is prescribed for subsequent treatment?
   - Name of the drug
   - Initial dose per day for the first two days for a 60 kg adult
   - Route of administration.

3 What test is used to monitor the effectiveness of treatment?

4 In the first five days, how often should this be checked?

5 For how long should treatment be given for this patient?

CASE
140

Answers

1 What form of drug therapy is used for the initial management?
   - *Name of the drug: low molecular weight heparin (Clexane®)*
   - *Approximate dose for a 60 kg patient: 90 mg (1.5 mg/kg)*
   - *Route of administration: subcutaneous*
   - *Frequency of treatment per day: once daily.*

2 What drug therapy is prescribed for subsequent treatment?
   - *Name of the drug: warfarin*
   - *Initial dose per day for the first two days for a 60 kg adult: 6–10 mg*
   - *Route of administration: oral.*

3 What test is used to monitor the effectiveness of treatment?
   International normalised ratio (INR).

4 In the first five days, how often should this be checked?
   Daily.

5 For how long should treatment be given for this patient?
   Three months.

CASE
140

CASE 141

Hypertension

Hypertension is a common medical condition that requires careful control with appropriate drug therapy.

Blood pressure is a function of cardiac output and peripheral resistance (BP = CO x PR), and cardiac output is a function of stroke volume and heart rate (CO = SV x HR). For each factor listed below, name one drug which causes it to be reduced and therefore decreases blood pressure. In addition to the name of the drug, give the usual dose for an adult patient and one important side effect. Name:

1 a drug that reduces peripheral resistance

2 a drug that reduces the heart rate

3 a drug that decreases stroke volume.

Therapeutics and pharmacology

Answers

Check individual student answers with the *British National Formulary –
antihypertensive drugs.*

eg drugs that reduce:

1 Peripheral resistance:
    • *Calcium channel blocking drugs*
    • *ACE inhibitors.*

2 Heart rate:
    • *Beta-blockers.*

3 Stroke volume:
    • *diuretic drugs*
    • *Beta-blockers.*

Therapeutics and pharmacology

CASE
141

CASE 142

Angina pectoris

A variety of drugs can be used to treat angina pectoris. What four drugs would you consider using if you needed to prescribe anti-anginal medication for a 75 kg man who has no other significant medical history and is on no other medication? Please list four drugs, each with a different mode of action, together with the dose, route of administration and dosage regime, and name one major side effect of which the patient needs to be informed.

Answers

Check individual student answers with the *British National Formulary*.

Drugs to be chosen from four of the following categories:

- *Aspirin/antiplatelet drugs*
- *Nitrates*
- *ß-Blockers*
- *Calcium-channel blockers*
- *Potassium-channel activators eg nicorandil.*

Therapeutics and pharmacology

CASE
142

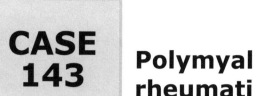

CASE 143

Polymyalgia rheumatica

A 65-year-old woman has been diagnosed as having polymyalgia rheumatica and requires long-term prednisolone therapy.

1 What investigation should be performed before this treatment is started or within the first few weeks of therapy?

2 List five of the major side effects of steroid therapy.

3 If this patient is also taking warfarin, what effect will starting prednisolone have on the international normalised ratio (INR)?

4 If the patient is taking non-steroidal anti-inflammatory analgesic drugs, what side effect or complication may develop?

5 What effect does steroid therapy have on the white blood cell count?

Answers

1 What investigation should be performed before this treatment is started or within the first few weeks of therapy?

   Bone density test.

2 List five of the major side effects of steroid therapy.
   - *Weight gain*
   - *Avascular necrosis*
   - *Reduced wound healing*
   - *Fluid retention*
   - *Cushing's syndrome*
   - *Psychosis*
   - *Hypertension*
   - *Increased risk of infection*
   - *Peptic ulceration*
   - *Diabetes*
   - *Adrenal suppression*
   - *Candida infection*
   - *Osteoporosis*
   - *Reactivation of tuberculosis*
   - *Hirsutism.*

3 If this patient is also taking warfarin, what effect will starting prednisolone have on the international normalised ratio (INR)?

   Reduces the INR.

4 If the patient is taking non-steroidal anti-inflammatory analgesic drugs, what side effect or complication may develop?

   Gastritis or peptic ulceration.

5 What effect does steroid therapy have on the white blood cell count?

   Increases the white cell count.

CASE
143

Index

systemic lupus erythematosus 39
sodium 88, 89, 91, 92
spastic paraparesis 68
splenomegaly 64
spontaneous pneumothorax 32
sputum production 5
sputum samples 34
steroids
   in psoriasis 37
   skin lesions 36
Stokes-Adams attacks 11
stomach, cancer 15
subcutaneous calcification 31
superior vena cava obstruction 33, 61
swollen legs 12, 52
syncopy 45
   ECG 103
systemic lupus erythematosus 24, 39
   clinical findings 67

telangiectasia 31
temporal arteritis 22
tension headache 22
thirst 20
thrombocytopenia 9, 36
thyrotoxicosis 14, 49, 98
tiredness 21
   ECG findings 101
tongue 46
total protein 88, 93
transient ischaemic attacks 11, 102
transient weakness 102
tuberculosis 76

ulcerative colitis 16, 40
urea 88, 89, 91, 92
urticaria 29

valvular dysfunction 77
ventricular ectopic beats 13
vertebrobasilar insufficiency 11
viral hepatitis 19
visual field assessment 71
vitamin B12 deficiency 86

ward observation chart
   bacteraemia 108
   gastrointestinal haemorrhage 106
   rising intracranial pressure 107
warfarin 36
weight loss 8, 14, 51, 78
   and loss of appetite 15
white cell count 87, 88, 92, 94

X-rays
   change in bowel habit 83
   chest pain and dyspnoea 76
   crampy abdominal pain 84
   dysphagia 82
   fever, cough and herpes labialis 70
   fever and haemoptysis 81
   gradually increasing dyspnoea 85
   increasing dyspnoea 77
   recurrent chest infections and weight loss 78
   recurrent pleuritic pains 80
xanthelasma 26

PASTEST BOOKS FOR MEDICAL STUDENTS

PasTest are the specialists in study guides and revision courses for medical qualifications. For over 30 years we have been helping doctors to achieve their potential. The PasTest range of books for medical students includes:

100 Clinical Cases and OSCEs in Medicine   1 904627 12 9
David McCluskey

100 Clinical Cases and OSCEs in Surgery   1 904627 00 5
Noel Aherne, Enda McDermott, Arnold D K Hill

OSCEs for Medical Students, 2nd edition, Volume 1   1 901198 04 9
Adam Feather, Ramanathan Visvanathan, John SP Lumley

OSCEs for Medical Students, 2nd edition, Volume 2   1 901198 05 7
Adam Feather, Ramanathan Visvanathan, John SP Lumley

OSCEs for Medical Students, 2nd edition, Volume 3   1 904627 11 0
Adam Feather, Ramanathan Visvanathan, John SP Lumley, Jonathan Round

EMQs for Medical Students Volume 1   1 901198 65 0
Adam Feather et al

EMQs for Medical Students Volume 2   1 901198 69 3
Adam Feather et al

EMQs for Medical Students: Practice Papers, Volume 3   1 904627 07 2
Adam Feather et al

Essential MCQs for Medical Finals, Second edition   1 901198 20 0
Rema Wasan, Delilah Hassanally, Balvinder Wasan

Essential MCQs for Surgical Finals, Second edition   1 901198 15 4
Delilah Hassanally, Rema Singh

Essential MCQs in Clinical Pharmacology   1 901198 32 4
Delilah Hassanally, Rema Singh

Essential MCQs in Obstetrics and Gynaecology   1 901198 34 0
Diana Hamilton-Fairley

Medical Finals: Passing the Clinical, 2nd edition   1 904627 63 4
Christopher Moore, Anne Richardson

Surgical Finals: Passing the Clinical, 2nd edition   1 901198 77 4
Gina Kuperberg, John SP Lumley

Medical Finals: Structured Answers and Essay Questions   0 906896 79 7
Adam Feather, Ramanathan Visvanathan, John SP Lumley

Surgical Finals: Structured Answers and Essay Questions, Second Edition
Ramanathan Visvanathan, John SP Lumley   1 901198 43 X

Learning by Lists for Medical Students   1 901198 30 8
Stuart McPherson

The Practical Guide to Medical Ethics and Law for Junior Doctors and Medical Students   1 901198 76 6
Chloe-Maryse Baxter, Mark Brennan, Yvette Coldicott

Radiology Casebook for Medical Students   1 901198 40 5
Rema Wasan, Alan Grundy, Richard Beese

Clinical Skills for Medical Students: A Hands-on Guide   1 901198 86 3
Ian Bickle, Paul Hamilton, David McCluskey, Barry Kelly

Delivery to your door

With a busy lifestyle, nobody enjoys walking to the shops for something that may or may not be in stock. Let us take the hassle and deliver direct to your door. We will dispatch your book within 24 hours of receiving your order.

How to Order:

www.pastest.co.uk

To order books safely and securely online, shop at our website.

Telephone: +44 (0)1565 752000 Fax: +44 (0)1565 650264

For priority mail order and have your credit card to hand when you call.

Write to us at:

PasTest Ltd
Haig Road
Parkgate Industrial Estate
Knutsford
WA16 8DX